First Edition

Medicine for Consumers

Gregory Billy, M.D.

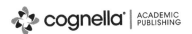

cognella® | ACADEMIC PUBLISHING

Bassim Hamadeh, CEO and Publisher

Gem Rabanera, Project Editor

Sean Adams, Production Editor

Jess Estrella, Senior Graphic Designer

Trey Soto, Licensing Coordinator

Natalie Piccotti, Director of Marketing

Kassie Graves, Vice President of Editorial

Jamie Giganti, Director of Academic Publishing

Cover copyright © Depositphotos/alexraths; © Depositphotos/Joingate; © Depositphotos/Icon_Craft_Studio; © Depositphotos/ibrandify.

Printed in the United States of America.

ISBN: 978-1-5165-2610-9 (pbk) / 978-1-5165-2611-6 (br)

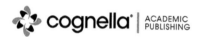

Brief Contents

Chapter 1 History of Medical Education   1

Chapter 2 Medical School   7

Chapter 3 Medical Training   13

Chapter 4 Inpatient Medicine   17

Chapter 5 Outpatient Medicine   25

Chapter 6 Medical Specialties   29

Chapter 7 Surgical Specialties   35

Chapter 8 Physician Office Visit   41

Chapter 9 The Pharmaceutical Industry   47

Chapter 10 Prescriptions and Medications   53

Chapter 11 Diagnostic Laboratory Tests   61

Chapter 12 Diagnostic Imaging Tests   67

Chapter 13 Dental Conditions   73

Chapter 14 Medical Diagnosis II   79

Chapter 15 Surgical Diagnosis II   87

Chapter 16 Nutrition Principles   93

Chapter 17	Nutrition Choices	101
Chapter 18	Exercise	107
Chapter 19	Complementary and Alternative Medicine	113
Chapter 20	Strength and Conditioning Coach	121
Chapter 21	Athletic Training	127
Chapter 22	Physical Therapy	131
Chapter 23	Occupational Therapy	137
Chapter 24	Speech-Language Pathologist	143
Chapter 25	Physician Assistant	149
Chapter 26	Psychologist	155
Chapter 27	Mental Health Issues	161
Chapter 28	Marijuana	169
Chapter 29	Sexually Transmitted Diseases	175
Chapter 30	Medicare and Medical Assistance	183
Chapter 31	Insurance Issues	193
Chapter 32	Electronic Medical Records	199
Chapter 33	Internet Searches	207
Chapter 34	Internet Claims	215
Chapter 35	Medical Myths	221

Chapter 36   International Travel   227

Chapter 37   Workers' Compensation   233

Chapter 38   Long-Term Care   241

Chapter 39   Advance Directives and End-of-Life Issues   247

Chapter 40   Patient Satisfaction   255

Chapter 41   Picking the Right Physician   261

Detailed Contents

Chapter 1   History of Medical Education   1
     History   1
     References   5

Chapter 2   Medical School   7
     Undergraduate Education   7
     Medical School   8
     Resources   12

Chapter 3   Medical Training   13
     Postgraduate Education   13
     Resources   16

Chapter 4   Inpatient Medicine   17
     Inpatient Care   17
     Reference   23
     Resources   23

Chapter 5   Outpatient Medicine   25
     Factors Impacting Delivery   25
     Competition   26
     Ambulatory Care Centers   26
     Reference   28

Chapter 6   Medical Specialties   29
     Decision   29

Chapter 7   Surgical Specialties   35
     Hierarchy?   35
     Second Opinion   35

Chapter 8   Physician Office Visit   41
     Office Visits   41
     Reference   45

Chapter 9   The Pharmaceutical Industry   47

      Industry   47

      Development   47

      Research   48

      Marketing   49

      References   51

      Resources   51

Chapter 10   Prescriptions and Medications   53

      Prescription   53

      Controlled Substances Act   54

      Drug Schedules   54

      Addiction   56

      Medications in Pregnancy   57

      Placebo   58

      Generic Medication   58

      Copay Structure   58

      Over-the-Counter Medications   58

      References   59

      Resource   59

Chapter 11   Diagnostic Laboratory Tests   61

      Diagnosis   61

      Resource   65

Chapter 12   Diagnostic Imaging Tests   67

      Diagnosis   67

      References   72

      Resource   72

Chapter 13   Dental Conditions   73

      Dentist   73

      Dental Hygienist   73

      Dental Assistant   74

      Dental Specialties   74

      Tooth Anatomy   74

      References   77

      Resources   78

Chapter 14 Medical Diagnosis II   79
          Introduction   79
          Gastroesophageal Reflux Disease   79
          Concussion   81
          Multiple Sclerosis   82
          References   84

Chapter 15 Surgical Diagnosis II   87
          Introduction   87
          Appendicitis   87
          Rotator Cuff Tendinitis   89
          Carpal Tunnel Syndrome   90
          References   92

Chapter 16 Nutrition Principles   93
          Nutrition   93
          Output   94
          Input   95
          References   98
          Resources   99

Chapter 17 Nutrition Choices   101
          Nutrition   101
          References   105
          Resource   105

Chapter 18 Exercise   107
          Exercise   107
          References   111
          Resources   112

Chapter 19 Complementary and Alternative Medicine   113
          Complementary Medicine   113
          Alternative Medicine   113
          References   119
          Resources   120

Chapter 20 Strength and Conditioning Coach   121
          Strength and Conditioning Coach   121
          Resources   125

Chapter 21   Athletic Training   127
     Athletic Trainers   127
     Resources   130

Chapter 22   Physical Therapy   131
     Physical Therapist   131
     Resources   135

Chapter 23   Occupational Therapy   137
     Occupational Therapist   137
     Resources   141

Chapter 24   Speech–Language Pathologist   143
     Speech–Language Pathologist   143
     Resources   147

Chapter 25   Physician Assistant   149
     Physician Assistant   149
     References   152
     Resources   152

Chapter 26   Psychologist   155
     Psychologist   155
     Resources   159

Chapter 27   Mental Health Issues   161
     Psychiatrist   161
     Psychologist   161
     Diagnostic and Statistical Manual of Mental Disorder   162
     References   166
     Resources   167

Chapter 28   Marijuana   169
     Recreational Drug Use   169
     Marijuana   169
     References   174
     Resources   174

Chapter 29   Sexually Transmitted Diseases   175
     Conditions   175
     Latex Condoms   175

	Gonorrhea	176
	Chlamydia	177
	HPV	178
	Genital Herpes	179
	HIV	180
	Syphilis	180
	References	182

Chapter 30   Medicare and Medical Assistance   183
                  Terms   183
                  History   183
                  Organization   185
                  Medicare Supplemental Insurance   189
                  Medicaid   189
                  References   190
                  Resources   191

Chapter 31   Insurance Issues   193
                  Premium   193
                  Deductible   193
                  Coinsurance   194
                  Allowed Amount   194
                  Consolidated Omnibus Budget Reconciliation Act   194
                  Copayment   194
                  Flexible Spending Account   195
                  Health Savings Accounts   195
                  Health Maintenance Organization   196
                  Preferred Provider Organization   196
                  Point of Service Plan   196
                  Insurance Issues   196

Chapter 32   Electronic Medical Records   199
                  Electronic Records   199
                  Paper Medical Chart   200
                  Conversion   202
                  Meaningful Use   203
                  References   205
                  Resources   205

Chapter 33 Internet Searches 207
    MEDLINE 207
    Research Studies 208
    Searches 211
    References 212
    Resources 212

Chapter 34 Internet Claims 215
    Innovation 215
    Physician Access 216
    Dr. Google 216
    Domains 217
    Health Sites 218
    False Claims 219
    References 220

Chapter 35 Medical Myths 221
    Urban Legend 221
    References 225

Chapter 36 International Travel 227
    International Travel 227
    Reference 231
    Resources 232

Chapter 37 Workers' Compensation 233
    History 233
    Workers' Compensation in the United States 235
    Occupational Safety and Health Act 236
    Work Injury 236
    Predictive Factors 238
    References 239
    Resource 240

Chapter 38 Long-Term Care 241
    Long-Term Care 241
    Types of Long-Term Care 242
    Costs 243
    Home Care Services 245
    Nursing Home Factors to Consider 245

| | References | 246 |
| | Resources | 246 |

Chapter 39 Advance Directives and End-of-Life Issues 247
	Terms	247
	References	253
	Resources	253

Chapter 40 Patient Satisfaction 255
	History	255
	Fee for Service	255
	Capitation	256
	Value-Based Purchasing	256
	Emphasis on Outcomes	258
	References	259
	Resources	259

Chapter 41 Picking the Right Physician 261
	Insurance	261
	Other Factors	261
	Board Certification	262
	Results	263
	Websites	263
	Online Resources	263
	Resources	264

History of Medical Education

Objective

> ▸ Basic understanding of the history and development of medical education in the United States

History

Medical Education

During the 1600s and 1700s, most colonial Americans intending to practice medicine would serve as an apprentice for an already established physician. In Europe, small groups of physicians would create proprietary medical schools.[1] The wealthy would travel to Europe, typically Great Britain, to receive training either at a proprietary school or hospital. The larger cities: London, Edinburgh, and Paris offered medical schools with the advantage of learning in these large hospitals. Others entered the medical profession more directly by establishing a reputation as a healer or by selling curatives.

During the mid- to late 1700s, medical schools were established in the United States. By 1820 there were 13 medical schools in the United States.[2] The first medical school in the country was the University of Pennsylvania. Schools then began to develop a curriculum; early training consisted of 8 to 10 months of class lectures followed by a period of serving as an apprentice, similar to the modern-day education of physicians. Toward the late 1800s medical schools developed a curriculum that was more rigorous, as medical knowledge expanded and became more grounded in science.[3]

Another major event that influenced the medical education system was the formation of what would become the American Medical Association (AMA) in 1846. The goals of the AMA included higher standards of education and practice. There was a power struggle following the formation of the AMA, among physician groups who promoted reform and those who opposed reform.

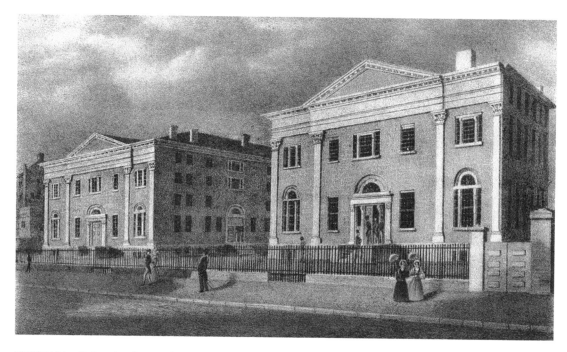

FIGURE 1.1   University of Pennsylvania, the first medical school in the United States.

Flexner Report

In 1910 Abraham Flexner, an educator and member of the research staff of the Carnegie Foundation, published a comprehensive report of the state of medical education in the United States and Canada. He surveyed all 155 medical and osteopathic educational institutions in the United States and Canada.

Flexner concluded that the education offered by medical institutions was substandard. His report concluded that there were too many institutions and that freestanding educational institutions were hard pressed to produce the funding necessary to maintain a quality level of education.

His report further recommended that medical schools have minimum admission standards, including a high school education and at least 2 years of studies at the college level. Additionally, the report recommended that medical schools should be 4 years in duration: 2 years of basic sciences and 2 years of clinical practice. "Proprietary" schools should be closed or incorporated into universities. As a result of the report, between 1910 and 1935 more than half of all American medical schools merged or closed. The majority of the affected schools were osteopathic schools.

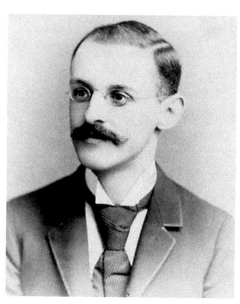

FIGURE 1.2   Abraham Flexner.

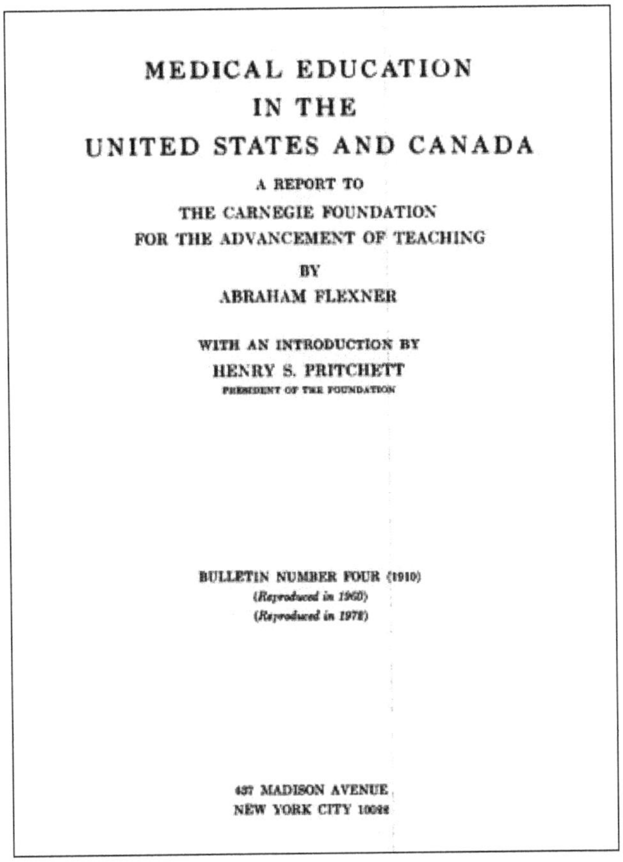

MEDICAL EDUCATION
IN THE
UNITED STATES AND CANADA

A REPORT TO
THE CARNEGIE FOUNDATION
FOR THE ADVANCEMENT OF TEACHING

BY
ABRAHAM FLEXNER

WITH AN INTRODUCTION BY
HENRY S. PRITCHETT
PRESIDENT OF THE FOUNDATION

BULLETIN NUMBER FOUR (1910)
(Reproduced in 1960)
(Reproduced in 1972)

437 MADISON AVENUE
NEW YORK CITY 10022

FIGURE 1.3   Flexner Report.

Of the 66 surviving medical schools in 1935, 57 were university based. Flexner was particularly impressed by Johns Hopkins Medical School and Hospital and thought it served as a model institution.

Another important factor driving the mergers and closures of medical schools was the fact that the AMA worked with the individual state medical boards to adopt and enforce the report's recommendations.

It is somewhat remarkable that more than 100 years later, the *Flexner Report* still serves as the basis for medical education in the United States today.

FACT TO KNOW

If asked, most Americans will identify the medical symbol as a caduceus. Below is a caduceus, which is typically mistaken for the symbol representing medicine.

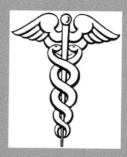

This is not the symbol for medicine, it is the symbol for commerce. Below is the symbol for medicine, the Rod of Asclepius.

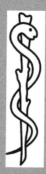

Why the confusion? The U.S. Army Medical Corps used the following symbol in the early 1900s.

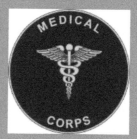

As you can see, it uses the caduceus. Most ambulances, however, are identified by the Rod of Asclepius.

References

1. Fee, E. The first American medical school: the formative years. *The Lancet*. Volume 385, Issue 9981, 1940–1.
2. Rothstein, W. G. (1987). *American Medical Schools and the Practice of Medicine: A History*. New York, NY: Oxford University Press; 1987.
3. Ludmerer, K. M. (1999). *Time to Heal: American Medical Education from the Turn of the Century to the Era of Managed Care*. New York: Oxford University Press, 1999.

Figure Credits

2

Medical School

Objectives

> ▸ Understanding of the process of applying to medical school, with emphasis on the competitive nature for admission
> ▸ Review of the classic medical school curriculum and education

Undergraduate Education

Medical schools are professional schools, and admission into the schools requires an undergraduate degree. The process of applying to medical school begins with choosing an undergraduate school. There are a multitude of factors to consider when choosing an undergraduate school, including but not limited to: cost, location, and reputation. Undergraduate schools will typically provide visiting prospective students with statistics concerning the schools' acceptance rate into graduate programs which include medical schools. These rates can vary widely, with some acceptance rates approaching 98%. Why such a variation? Some schools—more specifically the premed committee—will not support your application for medical school admission unless they are convinced that you will be accepted, thereby preserving their high acceptance rate. Other schools with lower acceptance rates will support your candidacy for admission with a less-than-stellar undergraduate academic record. Being aware of the prospective school's premed committee policy is an important factor to consider.

Another factor to consider is deciding between a small private undergraduate college versus a large public university. While a small private college may have a great academic reputation, its reputation may only be local or regional. The large public university will likely have a national reputation. This factor may help if you need to expand your medical school applications to a larger geographic area to include schools throughout the country.

Medical School

There are two subtypes of medical schools: allopathic and osteopathic. *Osteopathic* medical schools originated in and are unique to the United States. *Allopathic* schools will confer the doctor of medicine (MD) degree and the osteopathic schools the doctor of osteopathy (DO) degree. Allopathic schools have a more competitive admissions process than osteopathic schools. Graduates of either school are doctors who complete a 4-year medical education program. Both will be licensed physicians who can diagnose and perform surgeries. Allopathic graduates will be licensed after successfully passing the three-step United States Medical Licensure Examination (USMLE). The National Board of Osteopathic Medical Examiners administers a three-step examination COMLEX-USA to osteopathic graduates for licensure. The allopathic approach focuses on diagnosis and treatment based on patients' symptoms. The osteopathic approach is a holistic integrative approach. Osteopathic schools produce around 20% and allopathic schools about 80% of graduating physicians each year.

TABLE 2.1   MEDICAL SCHOOL APPLICATION COMPONENTS

Background information

Course work/transcripts

Work and activities

Letters of evaluation

Personal comments essay

MCAT examination scores

Application Process

Applying to medical school is done through the Association of American Medical Colleges (AAMC). The application process is completed online. The American Medical College Application Service® (AMCAS®) is the AAMC's centralized medical school application processing service. The 2018 AMCAS application fee is $160, which includes one medical school application; the cost is $39 for each additional medical school application. The application process is submitted online and consists of multiple sections (Table 2.1).

Application

The application requires submission of your college transcript(s) as well as the Medical College Admission Test (MCAT) scores. The MCAT is the medical school version of the SAT/ACT. The MCAT was updated in April 2015. It is a standardized, multiple-choice examination designed to assess knowledge of biological/biochemical, chemical/physical, psychological/social behavior, and critical thinking/reasoning skills. Scores are reported in these four sections, which consist of 53 to 59 questions each.

Another important component of the application is the personal essay. The essay is the candidate's opportunity to provide his or her perspective and desire to become a physician. It is the place for a candidate to explain what makes him or her unique compared to the other thousand applicants the committee is reviewing. The essay is limited to one page and serves as a true test to the candidate to remain relevant yet concise.

Response

After the application is reviewed by the medical school admission committee, the applicant will receive a decision. The response options are similar to when one asks another out on a date: yes or no. The school will either reject the applicant or invite him or her for an interview. The interview will be set up on a date that has been mutually agreed upon by the candidate and school.

Interview

The interview day usually occurs with a number of other prospective students. The medical school will provide the group of candidates with a tour of the medical campus, including classrooms, hospitals, outpatient centers, and clinics. The candidate will typically interview with two or three faculty members at the medical school. It is important for applicants to be themselves, be as comfortable as they can be, and be confident but not cocky. The candidates need to bring out what makes them a unique and good fit for that particular school. It is also important for candidates to be respectful to everyone during the application and interview process. Feedback is sometimes taken from everyone involved in the interview process, including administrative assistants, and not only the interviewing physicians.

Decision

After interviewing candidates at a particular program, the medical school will again render a decision. The decision is somewhat similar to the decision to grant an interview, although this time with an additional option. The school will either accept the candidate into its medical school, reject the candidate, or wait-list the candidate.

The rejection decision ends a prospective student's chance for admission at that medical school for the coming year. Rejected candidates may choose to reach out to the medical school's admission committee and ask how they can improve their chances of acceptance when reapplying to medical school in the future.

The accepted candidate may choose to accept the school's offer. This candidate may indeed have multiple offers of acceptance to consider. This is the principle behind the waitlist response to other applicants. By waitlisting, the school thinks strongly of a candidate's possible matriculation to the school but feels other candidates are better suited. Therefore, if the accepted candidate has multiple acceptances and chooses to attend another school, his or her place in the upcoming class will be filled by the next person on the wait list. The medical school may then be able to change a candidate's status from wait-listed to accepted.

Medical School

Medical schools consist of a 4-year program, outlined in Table 2.2. Traditionally, the first 2 years are spent in labs and lecture halls and the last 2 years in hospitals and clinics.

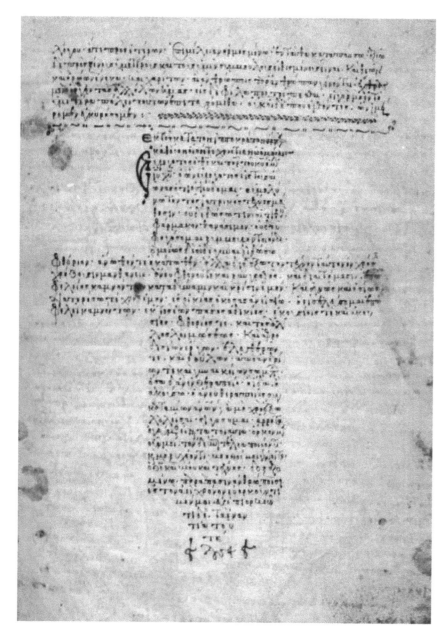

FIGURE 2.1   Hippocratic Oath

There has been a recent emphasis to increase students' clinical exposure during the first 2 years of school. During the first year the emphasis is on the study of anatomy, physiology, histology, and biochemistry. The second year emphasizes clinical sciences focusing on pathology, microbiology, and pharmacology. In the third year students will begin clinical rotations, spending time on the floors and assisting the medical team in evaluating patients and learning treatment approaches. Most clinical rotations will last between 4 and 8 weeks, giving students a broad exposure to the various disciplines of medicine. During the fourth and final year of medical school, students continue clinical rotations and have opportunities to do elective clinical rotations. The elective rotations are usually in areas that students would like to pursue in a postgraduate program or residency upon graduation from medical school. The entire 4-year experience can at times be both physically and emotionally challenging.

Graduation Day

After 4 years of medical school, students look forward to graduation day. During the graduation ceremony, students are conferred the degree of doctors. It is during this ceremony that the Hippocratic Oath is recited by the new physicians. The oath was written in antiquity. The new physician will practice to abide by its principles: treat the sick to the best of your ability, preserve patient privacy, and educate the next generation of physicians with the principles of medicine. Some physicians also like to add "do no harm to the patient." Although this is actually not in the written or recited in the oath; it is a principle that physicians will subscribe to.

TABLE 2.2   TRADITIONAL MEDICAL SCHOOL PROGRAM

Year 1	basic sciences: anatomy, physiology, histology, biochemistry
Year 2	clinical sciences: pathology, microbiology, pharmacology
Year 3	clinical rotations: medicine, pediatrics, surgery, OB–GYN
Year 4	clinical rotations: neurology, emergency medicine, and clinical electives

FACT TO KNOW

Getting accepted into medical school is quite competitive, and the number of applicants for a select number of slots is significant. At first glance the statistics can seem incredibly daunting. For example, the Pennsylvania State University College of Medicine recently received 9,449 applications for only 149 slots. This, mathematically, is a 1.57% matriculation rate. However, keep in mind that the average number of schools that an applicant applies to is 14. So that means if one is accepted, the applicant can only attend 1/14, which equates to a percentage of 7%. According to the most recent AAMC data, the overall acceptance rate is 32%. If it is your dream to be a physician, do not let the statistics overwhelm you.

Resources

American Association of Colleges of Osteopathic Medicine—website for osteopathic (DO) physicians. This site serves as a central site for application to osteopathic medical schools, education of the public and a resource for osteopathic physicians: http://www.aacom.org/

Association of American Medical Colleges—website for allopathic (MD) physicians. This site serves as a central site for application to allopathic medical schools, its members are all 151 accredited U.S. and 17 accredited Canadian medical schools; nearly all major teaching hospitals and health systems. It serves as a resource for those considering applying to medical school: http://www.aamc.org/

National Board of Osteopathic Medical Examiners—website of the national credentialing examination of osteopathic physicians. This site contains information of the testing and administration of the COMLEX-USA, certification examination: http://www.nbome.org

United States Medical Licensure Examination—website of the national credentialing examination of allopathic physicians. This site contains information of the testing and administration of the USMLE, the test for medical licensure in the United States: http://www.usmle.org/

Figure Credit

Fig. 2.1: Source: https://commons.wikimedia.org/wiki/File:HippocraticOath.jpg.

3

Medical Training

Objective

► Basic understanding of the postgraduate training of doctors, including work demands, experiences, and duration

Postgraduate Education

During their fourth and final year of medical school, prospective doctors will begin applying for postgraduate training positions. These positions are known as internships and residencies. All medical students receive very similar training during their four years of medical school. Students will experience similar exposures to different areas of medicine during their third- and fourth-year clinical rotations. The different skills of a physician are mastered during their training after medical school. Internships and residencies are the time when physicians gravitate toward a particular medical specialty. What influences which specialty a physician will further train in? Sometimes it is a unique medical student–patient experience that influences which specialty one will chose. Often the specialty may be influenced by a particular instructor–attending physician or senior resident that may influence the medical student. Other times the specialty may be influenced by a family member who is a physician. Certain specialties are more suited to a certain personality type. It is during residency training that different postgraduate skills will emerge and physicians will specialize into various fields.

The Match

Fourth-year medical students will apply to different residency programs, similar to the process of applying to medical schools. The residency program may grant them an interview based on their medical school transcripts, national board scores (USMLE or COMLEX-USA), and letters of recommendation from current medical school professors. The interviews will be scheduled between the medical students and the prospective residency program. The interviews are similar to the medical school interview. The different training programs will provide prospective residents with a tour of the facility highlighting the positive and unique aspects of their training program. Larger academic and teaching hospitals will have more slots for residents as well as a larger variety of programs. The programs may also be staffed by leading physicians in their particular field. Smaller hospitals with fewer total positions may offer a better opportunity for more hands-on training opportunities. For example, neurologic problems in a larger training program will be seen by a neurology resident or service, while at a smaller hospital these patients would be cared for by the internal medicine resident. Medical students will need to determine which program is best for them based on reputation, training, and location.

After interviewing at a number of residency training programs at their own expense, medical students will then make a list of these programs and rank them in order of preference, based on their desire to train at each particular program. For a nominal fee, students will submit their rank list to the National Resident Matching Program (the Match). The residency programs will also rank medical students based on their preferences and provide their rank lists to the Match.

Match Day
The rank lists are submitted by both groups in January and February, the results are revealed during match day. Typically in mid-March, medical students will be able to check the status of their match and find out if they matched a program they had ranked. If they did not match, they will be able to get a list of programs that did not fill their slots and work on contacting those programs for a residency position. This process is known as the "scramble."

The medical schools will likely have a match day celebration. All medical students will be together and be given an envelope containing their match program. The students will open the letter at the same time to learn of their future destinations. This is another milestone in the education of a physician. It is a unique event, since the soon-to-be physicians will then know the direction for their life for the next 3 to 7 years. The match results often contain surprises that can be both positive and negative.

Most medical schools will provide statistics about their successes with the match. The schools typically promote statistics stating that 80% of medical students will match at one of their top three choices. This may seem very successful, but there may be a big difference between your first and third choices, much like getting a bronze medal instead of a gold one. It is also important to keep in mind that certain specialties can be very competitive, and candidates who do not feel that they will match in a very competitive specialty may choose another specialty that they are more likely to match in.

Internship

Following medical school, newly graduated physicians will enter a residency program. Certain residencies that are specialized will have physicians do a year of *internship* training. Other training programs will not have the physician do an internship, also known as postgraduate year 1 (PGY-1). The internship is also known as a transitional or preliminary year. Internships offer a broad exposure to the different aspects of internal medicine or to the different aspects of surgery. Physicians are paid during their internship. This also marks the first time that new doctors are responsible for patient care; they do, however, provide care in a team structure.

Residency

Training programs to provide physicians with more specialized training in certain subspecialties are known as *residencies*. They can vary in length and are listed in Table 3.1. Residency programs are accredited by the Accreditation Council for Graduate Medical Education (ACGME), a private organization that sets the standards for graduate medical programs in the United States. The ACGME ensures the programs meet the quality standards of the specialty. Residency training is intense and the hours can be incredibly long. Since 2003 there have been restrictions limiting the number of work hours per week and per shift. Currently, the workweek is capped at 80 hours. First-year residents are not permitted to work more than a 16-hour shift, but this will likely be increased to a 24-hour shift similar to the limits for other residents. The limits are in place for both patient and resident safety concerns.

During residency training the resident physician will work in a team structure. The team will likely include an intern, junior resident, senior resident and an attending physician. The responsibilities of the resident will increase with their years of training or training level. According to the American Association of Medical Colleges, the starting median salary of a first year resident or intern is about $53,500. The salaries will typically increase by about $2,000 for each additional year of residency training.

TABLE 3.1   LENGTH OF RESIDENCY TRAINING

Years	Program
3	Family medicine, internal medicine, pediatrics, and emergency medicine
4	Obstetrics and gynecology, pathology, and psychiatry
3 plus PGY-1	Anesthesiology, dermatology, neurology, ophthalmology, and physical medicine and rehabilitation
4 plus PGY-1	Radiology and radiation oncology
5	General surgery, orthopedic surgery, otolaryngology, and plastic surgery
6	Neurological surgery

Legislature was recently passed to limit the number of hours that interns and residents work. Following residency, physicians will typically choose either to enter practice or subspecialize further by completing a fellowship.

Fellowship

Following residency, physicians may choose to subspecialize in their field by completing a *fellowship*. Fellowships are typically an additional 1 to 2 years of training. Examples include: an interventional fellowship in cardiology to get additional training and experience with cardiac catheterizations, a sports medicine fellowship for family practice residents who want to tailor their future practice toward athletic medicine, or a Micrographic Surgery and Dermatologic Oncology Fellowship in dermatology to gain additional experience in melanoma removal. Not all physicians will choose to do fellowships, as this will add another 1 to 2 years to their extensive training. The overall timeline is outlined in Table 3.2.

TABLE 3.2   PHYSICIAN EDUCATIONAL TIMELINE

College	Medical school	Internship (If not included in residency)	Residency	Fellowship	Total Years
4	4	(1)	3–6	1–2	11–16

FACT TO KNOW

The calendar year begins on January 1 and the fiscal year on October 1. When does the medical year begin? The medical year typically begins on July 1. This is the date that newly graduated physicians will start their internship or PGY-1, or the date when third-year residents becomes fourth-year residents, and so forth. Therefore, July 1 may not be the best time to schedule an elective medical procedure. The experience of residents will peak in the month of June and nadir in the month of July.

Resources

Accreditation Council for Graduate Medical Education—This website of the home site for ACGME, they accredit residency and fellowship programs to ensure academic standards: http://www.acgme.org

National Resident Matching Program—Home of the residency match program, when and where to apply and details of the match process are answered at this site: http://www.nrmp.org

Association of American Medical Colleges—Home of the academic oversight of medical schools and major teaching hospitals, below is the link to specific resident physician salaries: https://www.aamc.org/data/stipend/

4

Inpatient Medicine

Objectives

- ► Review of the history of the hospital in the United States
- ► Basic understanding of the inpatient setting for medical care of patients
- ► Options for inpatient care

Inpatient Care

Inpatient care is care given to a patient who is admitted to a hospital, mental/behavioral health unit, nursing home, extended care facility, or other medical facility and who stays overnight or greater than 24 hours in such a facility.

History of Hospitals in the United States

Currently, we take medical care for granted in our country. There are very likely choices to make between competing medical centers, and most medical

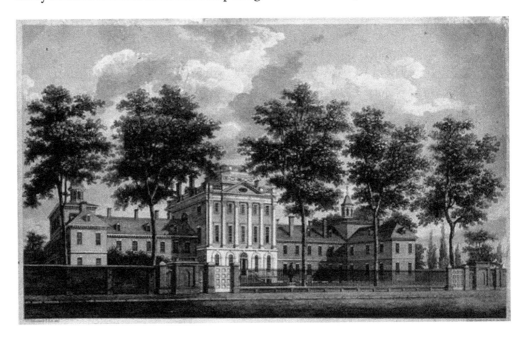

FIGURE 4.1   First hospital in the United States.

facilities are a few minutes away and easily accessible. This was not always the case; a little over 200 years ago, there were only two hospitals in the United States. The first hospital was in Philadelphia, founded in 1755, followed by New York Hospital in 1771.

By 1873 the United States had fewer than 180 hospitals, with a total of less than 50,000 beds. Even though the number of hospitals was increasing, the care they provided was not similar to today's standards, in both technology and outcomes. Early hospitals were not well organized and had little to offer in terms of specialty care. Most early hospitals only offered operating rooms for surgery, with most procedures being directed toward fracture reductions and care. Medicine at this time also had little to no understanding of infection, and diseases would spread quickly among patients. Additionally, physicians were neither affiliated nor integrated with hospitals, as they are today. Physicians would administer their care at the home of the patient, providing house calls. Technology was limited, and the early instruments of the physician were portable and carried in a doctor's bag.

Joseph Lister

A significant factor that advanced health care was our understanding of infection. In the late 19th century, Joseph Lister noted that nearly 50% of amputation patients died from sepsis. A few years later he learned of Louis Pasteur's theory of infections caused by microorganisms. Lister began using carbolic acid as an antiseptic to reduce bacterial contamination and was able to reduce the mortality rate in his surgical unit to 15%. This significantly improved the care that was being provided at hospitals.

The Civil War

Another factor that helped bring significant improvements in the American hospital system was the Civil War. The war was costly to our country in both injuries and casualties. Given the significant number of injuries and the desire to get the injured soldiers back to the fronts, hospitals needed to improve both their care and organization. Hospital care needed upgrading both north and south of the Mason–Dixon Line.

Mayo Clinic

In 1863, Dr. William Worrall Mayo moved to Rochester, Minnesota, to examine new recruits for the Union army. He stayed to set up a solo medical practice. His two sons, William J. and Charles H., joined him in practice after they finished medical school in the 1880s. Their first partner was added to the Mayo family practice in 1892. More physicians were invited to join the practice. The Mayo family practice became the first medical group practice. This type of partnership formed the concept of medical teamwork. Today the Mayo Clinic is the largest integrated, nonprofit medical group practice in the world. Doctors from every medical specialty work together to care for patients who come from all over the world for medical care and treatment.

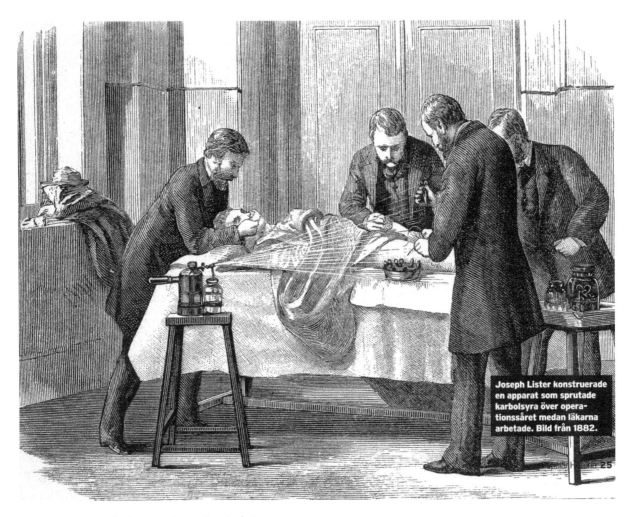

Joseph Lister konstruerade en apparat som sprutade karbolsyra över opera-tionssåret medan läkarna arbetade. Bild från 1882.

FIGURE 4.2   Joseph Lister spraying antiseptic during a surgery.

Hospitals continued to improve, and the relationship with physicians also changed. By the late 1800s, hospitals became essential to the practice of medicine and physicians. Technologies and outcomes improved significantly, and physicians began associating with hospitals. They began to admit their patients to hospitals for care. Physicians would follow the patients in the hospital for better outcomes, rather than solely providing home visits.

Florence Nightingale

Paramount to receiving better care in the hospital was the care provided by the nurses during a patient's stay. Nursing was unspecialized in the mid-1800s. There were not standards for education or certification. Hospitals may have been staffed by caring individuals, but the modern-day standards of nursing did not exist. Florence Nightingale initiated the first nursing school at St. Thomas' Hospital in London. The nursing school would address educational and professional standards that are in place today.

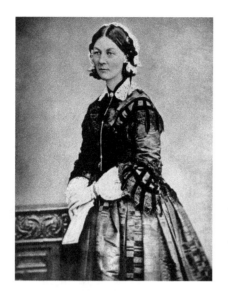

FIGURE 4.3   Florence Nightingale.

Today's nurses are highly educated and licensed to provide care to patients. The majority of which work in a hospital environment. One can become a nurse via three pathways: Bachelor of Science degree in nursing (BSN), Associate's degree in nursing (ADN) or obtaining a diploma from an approved nursing program. The BSN is obtained following completion of a four year program, this degree is felt necessary for administrative, teaching and research positions. The ADN entails a two- to three-year learning program. A nurse with an ADN degree may wish to further their education and go back to school via a RN-to-BSN program. The tuition associated with this program may frequently be offered as incentive benefit of the nurse's current employer. Some profession nurses may choose to attain additional training and work as nurse anesthetists, nurse practitioners or nurse midwives.

Registered nurses (RN) must be licensed. In order to become licensed, they must graduate from an approved program and pass the National Council Licensure Examination (NCLEX-RN).

According to the U.S. Department of Labor, the job outlook for nurses is projected to grow 15% from 2016 to 2026. The department also notes that the median annual wage for hospital-based nurses was $ 72,070 in May 2017.

Admission to a Hospital

Patients are admitted to a hospital in one of three ways: after evaluation in the emergency room (ER), by direct admission from a physician's office or outpatient clinic, or via transfer from another hospital or medical facility. See Table 4.1.

For admission to the hospital for care, certain criteria need to be met. These include: failure to respond to outpatient treatment, with worsening of the patient's clinical condition. Another reason for admission is that the current treatment plan will continue to be modified, and such changes to the treatment program are best done in an inpatient hospital setting. The most common reason is an abrupt change in medical status, including but not limited to chest pain, mental status changes, and new onset of neurologic deficits. Additionally, the patient may be admitted to the hospital after a 23-hour period of observation in the ER, where the condition is not expected to improve.

TABLE 4.1   ADMISSION TO A HOSPITAL

After evaluation in the ER

By direct admission from a physician's office or outpatient clinic
Via transfer from another hospital or medical facility

Physician Orders

Patients who are admitted to a hospital are usually admitted under the care or service of a physician or physician group. The admitting physician is responsible for supervising and ordering the care for the patient. What orders are typically written by the admitting or attending physician? The attending physician will order every aspect of the patient's care. See Table 4.2. The initial order is the admit order; the physician will provide the order to initiate admission to the hospital and then the level of care at the hospital. The level of care can range from an intensive care unit, regular floor, operating room, or behavioral health unit. Any pertinent precautions will also be outlined; these may include fall risks, seizure precautions, or non-weight bearing to any extremity recovering from a fracture. Vital signs, which are obtained by the nursing staff, include the patient's temperature, heart rate, breathing or respiration rate, and blood pressure. These will be ordered at specific frequencies, more frequent for unstable or critical patients and less frequent for more medically stable patients. The frequency of the vital signs can

TABLE 4.2 PHYSICIAN ORDERS
Admit
Unit
Precautions
Vital signs
Activity
IV
Diet
Allergies
Medications
Labs
Consults
Diagnostic tests

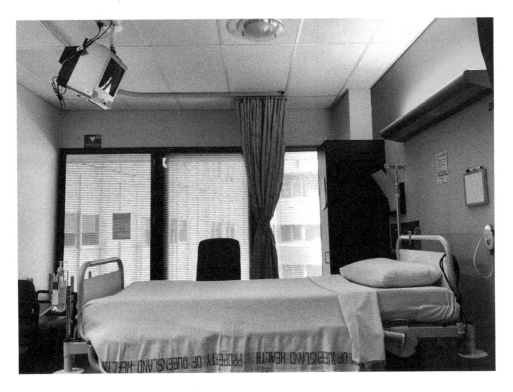

FIGURE 4.4   Typical inpatient hospital room.

range from every 15 minutes to daily. Activity will also be addressed by denoting bed rest, out of bed (OOB) with supervision, or ad lib (as able). Patients unable to drink enough fluid may require intravenous (IV) supplementation. The patient's diet will also be ordered and may include low sodium for patients with high blood pressure, cardiac diet low in saturated fats for patients with cardiac concerns, or a pureed diet with thickened liquids for patients following a stroke that has affected their ability to swallow. Any allergies will also need to be noted in the orders to prevent patients from receiving a medication that could cause a significant reaction or an anaphylactic (life-threatening) reaction. Likewise, any medications that the patient should or will need to take will be outlined in the order. Consults for physicians in different specialties may also be ordered for their input to help with the care of the patient. Any lab or diagnostic tests such as: X-rays, computerized tomography (CT) scans, electrocardiograms (EKGs), or magnetic resonance imaging (MRI) scans will also be ordered by the attending physician.

It is important for family members to remember to check with the nursing staff to know of any activity precautions or dietary concerns that may be ordered for loved ones during their stay in the hospital. Knowing any patient precautions or limitations concerning activity or diet can help prevent complications that may arise.

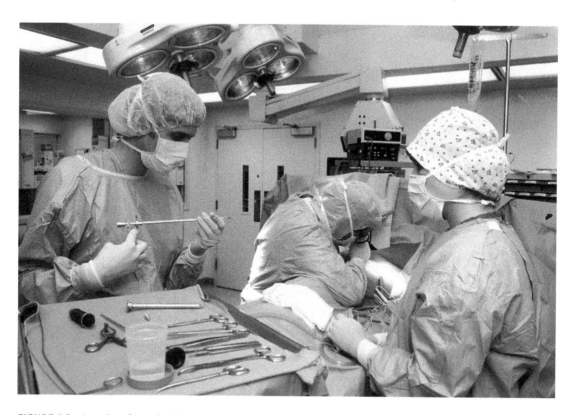

FIGURE 4.5   Inpatient Operating Room.

Reference

1. Vallbona, C., & Richards, T. (1999). Evolution of magnetic therapy from alternative to traditional medicine. *Physical Medicine and Rehabilitation Clinics of North America, 10*(3), 729–754.

Resources

Bureau of Labor Statistics—Site that details and overview of the profession, education, environment, pay and additional details of the nursing profession: https://www.bls.gov/ooh/healthcare/registered-nurses .htm#tab-1H20.

Council on Chiropractic Education—: National agency that promotes and oversees chiropractic education including accreditation of schools and training programs: http://cce-usa.org/

National Center for Complementary and Integrative Health—NIH sponsored sites that provides answers to all topics A-Z in complementary medicine, consumer friendly site: https://nccih.nih.gov/

Figure Credits

5

Outpatient Medicine

Objective

▸ Basic understanding of the outpatient setting for medical care of patients

Definition

▸ Care provided for a patient who is not hospitalized overnight but who visits a hospital, clinic, or associated facility for diagnosis or treatment.

Factors Impacting Delivery

Historically, health care procedures such as treatments and surgeries were done in a hospital environment. There has been a significant increase and emphasis on outpatient services over the past 20 years. Curtailing escalating costs have been the main factor in transitioning from an inpatient medical focus to the outpatient setting. The creation of Medicare in 1966 expanded the number of insured Americans, thereby increasing the use of services and subsequently the costs. With greater covered lives comes higher costs. Technology has also played a significant role, as new technologies are also associated with greater costs. These technologies include transplant surgeries, cardiac surgeries, and orthopedic joint replacements, all of which have become more common since the 1980s and 1990s, further increasing the costs of medical coverage.

The government and insurers have responded to the increase in medical costs across multiple fronts. There has been a significant decrease in inpatient services driven by the prospective payment system and managed care. This has let the shift toward outpatient treatment centers. These centers are commonly known as ambulatory care centers. *Ambulatory* indicates walking and is consistent with a certain degree of health. *Care* is synonymous with "treatment," while *center* is suggestive of a setting of excellence incorporating advanced technologies.

Outpatient services are cost effective. The associated costs are less than in a hospital setting, as outpatient service centers do not require an overnight stay. In addition, outpatient service centers usually specialize in one type of treatment or procedure. By specializing in a certain procedure day after day, this repetitive exposure will give the staff a lot of experience that is focused on the procedure the patient needs. Outpatient centers are better suited to deal with any complications if they perform thousands of procedures per year, versus a center that may only perform a few a week. Specialization should also allow the center to acquire the most advanced equipment and perform the latest techniques, both of which will produce improved outcomes and patient satisfaction.

Another patient convenience associated with outpatient services is that all care is provided in one place. All of the care that a patient needs before, during, and after the procedure, surgery, or test may be conveniently provided under one roof. Given the increase in ambulatory care centers over the past 2 decades, most people should be able to find a center that is both close and convenient to receive care.

Competition

Outpatient centers are profitable. Hospitals have little margin regarding inpatient care, while outpatient centers receive nice reimbursements for the care provided. The outpatient centers' actual costs show little variation, given the repetitive nature of the procedures being performed. The potential for profits has led to the proliferation of many ambulatory care centers. These centers may be owned by a hospital, health care plan, or privately by a medical group.

What factors are involved when choosing an ambulatory care center? Most patients will feel more comfortable in the care of a particular physician rather than a certain center. It may be best to pick a physician first, rather than an ambulatory care center, as the physician may not perform surgeries or procedures at the center. Choosing a center will also depend on one's insurance plan. Patient's may wish to utilize an outpatient center that is designated as a preferred or in plan center with their insurance plan.

Ambulatory Care Centers

The list of procedures and surgeries that can be performed at a surgical center is extensive. The APG Ambulatory Surgery Procedure List is approximately 75 printed pages long. These surgeries may include, but by no means are limited to, partial breast mastectomy, arthroscopic procedures of various joints, repair of nasal septum, and artery bypass grafting. It is more likely a surgery can be done at an ambulatory care center than not (see Table 5.1 for types of ambulatory care centers). Still, some surgeries are done in the hospital and require overnight stays, including joint replacements, surgery involving major organs, and the majority of spinal procedures.

Imaging centers are another example of an ambulatory care center. These centers specialize in imaging of the body both for diagnosis and treatment. These centers will typically be anchored by MRI. Studies to evaluate body structures by use of an MRI can confirm a patient's diagnosis and assist in directing treatments. In addition, some centers offer radiographic guided therapeutic procedures. Examples may include using imaging to place stents or assist with vertebroplasty (using cement at the site of a spinal compression fracture to provide stability and reduce pain).

Laboratory centers specialize in drawing and processing lab specimens and tests. The blood can be drawn and results run on a sample taken. Such centers will have experienced phlebotomists, individuals who draw blood samples on patients. Compared to a hospital, laboratory centers are usually a very convenient place to have blood drawn.

Gastrointestinal centers, which may provide screening or other services such as colonoscopy and endoscopy, are also becoming more common. These centers will specialize in procedures to evaluate the upper gastrointestinal (GI) tract (endoscopy) or the lower GI tract and rectum (colonoscopy). Such centers will perform thousands of these studies in a year and will become very proficient in this area.

In addition, physical therapy centers are another example of an ambulatory care center. Therapy centers will be staffed by a number of physical therapists. Given the number of physical therapists on-site, such centers have a greater likelihood of having certain therapists subspecialize. These subspecializations may include back pain, lymphedema (swelling of an extremity), stroke, and spinal cord injury.

Ambulatory care centers continue to be convenient centers for providing and administering medical care and treatments and likely will continue to play a significant role in health care delivery in the future.

TABLE 5.1 TYPES OF AMBULATORY CARE CENTERS
Surgery centers
Imaging centers
Cardiac catheterization centers
Mental or behavioral health centers
Substance abuse centers
Lab centers
Gastrointestinal centers
Durable medical equipment centers
Physical therapy centers
Chemotherapy and radiation therapy centers

NEED TO KNOW

Medicare may reimburse physicians at different rates for the same services, based on the location of the service. For example, compare a procedure performed at three different patient settings: a physician's office, a hospital outpatient department, and an ambulatory surgery center. The amount a physician was paid in 2013 for performing an epidural injection was $211.96 in a physician's office, $407.28 in an ambulatory surgery center, and $655.62 in a hospital outpatient department. The different reimbursement rates can really influence the location of care.[1]

Reference

1. Manchikanti, L., Benyamin, R. M., Falco, F. J., Hirsch, J. A. (2013). Recommendations of the Medicare Payment Advisory Commission (MEDPAC) on the health care delivery system: The impact on interventional pain management in 2014 and beyond. *Pain Physician, 6*(5), 419–440.

6

Medical Specialties

Objectives

- ▸ Basic understanding of the different medical primary specialties and subspecialties
- ▸ Idea of what is in a specialist's scope of practice

Definitions

- ▸ *Specialist:* A physician who specializes during residency training or does an additional fellowship.
- ▸ *Generalist:* A physician who is broadly trained in primary care services, including family physicians, internists, and pediatricians.

Decision

Choosing a specialty is typically done in the third year of medical school. The decision to pick a specific area of medicine may be related to the experiences the physician in training has during a particular rotation in medical school. The personality of the medical student is another determinant in choosing a particular medical specialty. Some future doctors prefer cerebral thinking and problem solving, while others (future surgeons) may enjoy working with their hands to fix something. Lastly, the lifestyle of the different specialties will also play an important factor. The ER physician may enjoy the unpredictability and the acute nature of the specialty, while the dermatologist may welcome the regular working hours with fewer on-call issues and emergency issues to address. Former athletes may gravitate toward an orthopedic surgery residency training program.

Family Physician

A family practice physician is a generalist who completes a residency training program of 3 years is a family physician. The family physician is trained to take care of the entire family, including children and adults. Training can also involve gynecology and obstetrics. Depending on geographic location, the family physician may care for pregnant patients and deliver babies. Family physicians may also be known as primary care physicians (PCPs) or "gatekeepers." This term refers to their role with certain insurance programs to provide necessary referrals for their patients to various specialties. They are typically involved with the initial workup of the patient. This initial workup may involve ordering various diagnostic tests and referrals to specialists if treatments are beyond their scope of practice. Recently, the position of PCP is moving more towards an outpatient practice, with less inpatient coverage of admitted patients.

Internist

An *internist* is another example of a generalist. Internists complete a 3-year residency program. Their training will focus on the care of adults. They also serve as a PCP and will begin the initial workup of a patient. They refer less to a specialist and initiate the treatment for common diseases and problems. Historically, internists have admitted their patients to hospitals for necessary care. There has been a shift toward an exclusive outpatient practice. Their patients are still admitted to a hospital but may be followed by a hospitalist—a physician trained in taking care of hospitalized patients. Hospitalists may cover the patient in the intensive care unit, telemetry unit, or regular medical floor. They frequently work 12-hour shifts caring for their patients.

Pediatrician

Pediatricians are generalists who are trained in the care of children. Pediatricians classically care for patients under age 18. Care for a child is distinctly different than caring for an adult. Children have different medical issues and problems than adults, and their treatments also differ in both approach and dosing of medications. Pediatricians become well trained in both diagnosing and treating diseases unique to children. Caring for sick children can be an emotionally trying experience. Seeing a sick or ill child can be quite sobering, and it requires the physician to have a certain personality type. Further complicating children's care may be their inability to speak or to appropriately communicate their symptoms. Difficult parents can present additional challenges. The length of training is 3 years, and various fellowships are available to further subspecialize.

Specialists

Specialists are typically named according to their field of study. *Ologist* is a suffix that typically denotes a particular field of science or an expert. The field of study is the prefix. Examples are listed in Table 6.1.

Cardiologist

A cardiologist is a specialist who treats the heart and heart-related problems. Cardiologists first complete a 3-year internal medicine residency and then a 3-year cardiology fellowship. During the fellowship training, they learn to manage various heart-related issues, including coronary artery disease, heart failure, or irregular heart rates known as arrhythmias. Some may choose to get additional training and subspecialize further by doing a second subspecialty fellowship for an additional 2 years. The subspecialty training is offered in cardiac catheterizations, heart failure, and heart arrhythmias. Based on their training, cardiologists can treat patients either noninvasively or invasively.

Noninvasive cardiologists will focus on the medical management of cardiovascular disease, prescribing medications to help reduce heart-related problems. Invasive cardiologists will be proficient in procedures to treat heart disease. These procedures include cardiac catheterizations and pacemaker implantation. The cardiac catherization is a procedure that involves injecting dye in the arteries and evaluating the flow pattern of the arteries (coronary) that provide blood to the heart. Once the blockages have been identified the cardiologist can use a balloon to place a metal stent to restore flow to the various vessels of the heart.

TABLE 6.1   COMMON SPECIALTIES

Cardio: heart

Derm: skin

Endo: glands

Gastro: stomach/digestive tract

Neuro: brain and nerves

Opthalmo: eyes

Pulmo: lungs

Path: disease

Pulmonologist

Pulmonologists are specialists who treat lung and breathing-related issues. They will complete a 3-year internal medicine residency and then a 2-year pulmonary fellowship. During the fellowship years, they learn to manage respiratory-related conditions. Common lung conditions include asthma, chronic obstructive pulmonary disease (COPD), and infections of the lungs. Pulmonologists will also perform and interpret pulmonary function tests to better understand the capacity and function of the lungs as well as prescribe medications and inhalers to improve breathing.

Pulmonologists will also perform bronchoscopies. A bronchoscopy involves inserting a flexible tube and camera into the trachea (windpipe) and viewing the bronchus and proximal lung tissues. During this procedure, a tissue sample, or biopsy, may be done to investigate a mass in this area.

Nephrologists

Nephrologists are specialists who treat diseases related to the kidneys. They complete a 3-year internal medicine residency and then complete a 2- to 3-year nephrology

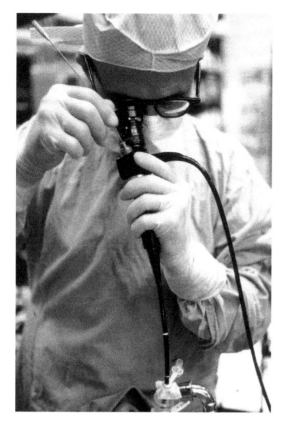

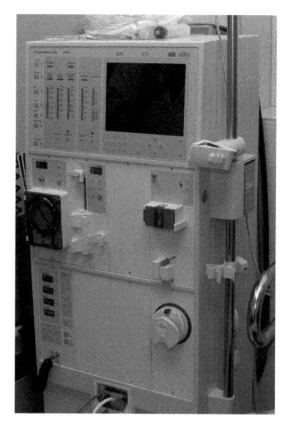

FIGURE 6.1   Pulmonologist performing a bronchoscopy.

FIGURE 6.2   Example of a hemodialysis machine.

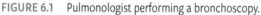

fellowship. Diseases of the kidney and kidney failure are the main focus of nephrologists. They will also manage dialysis treatments for patients in renal or kidney failure.

Endocrinologists

Endocrinologists are specialists who treat diseases related to the glands of the body. They complete a 3-year internal medicine residency and then complete a 2- to 3-year endocrinology fellowship. The fellowship focuses on the diagnosis and treatment of hormone disorders and imbalances caused by endocrine glands. The most commonly treated condition is the control of elevated blood glucoses (sugars) know as diabetes mellitus. The development of type 2 diabetes is closely related to obesity and unfortunately has been on the rise in the United States over the past 2 decades and responsible for significant morbidity and mortality.

Gastroenterologists

Gastroenterologists are specialists who treat diseases related to the digestive system (from the mouth to the rectum). Gastroenterologists complete a 3-year internal medicine residency and then a 3-year fellowship. The fellowship emphasizes subspecialty training in diseases of the GI tract. During this time gastroenterologists become proficient in performing invasive procedures to directly view the lining of the GI tract. One procedure is the endoscopy, an invasive procedure to view the esophagus and stomach. Another is the colonoscopy, an invasive procedure to view the rectum and large intestine. The procedures are done to evaluate the presence of masses or tumors as well as areas of bleeding. Gastroenterologists will also medically treat inflammatory issues of the bowels and heartburn or reflux issues.

Neurologist
Neurologists are physicians who specialize in the treatment of diseases related to the nervous system. They complete a 4-year residency, during which their training focuses on diagnosing and treating diseases of the central nervous system (brain and spinal cord) and the peripheral nervous system (nerves of the body). Neurologists perform procedures such as electrodiagnostic studies (nerve and muscle tests), electroencephalogram (EEG) studies, and sleep studies. In addition, they will also medically manage the diseases of the central nervous system: Parkinson's disease, seizures, and multiple sclerosis.

Psychiatrists
Psychiatrists are physicians who specialize in the diagnosis and treatment of mental disorders. They complete a 4-year residency, during which the focus of their training is to evaluate patients to determine whether their symptoms are the result of a physical illness, a combination of physical and mental, or a strictly psychiatric one. Psychiatrists can easily subspecialize in various areas, including addiction disorders, child and adolescent psychiatry, geriatric psychiatry, and forensic psychiatry. Psychiatrists may work closely with counselors and psychologists to help treat patients. The main difference between a psychiatrist and a psychologist is the former is a medical doctor who can prescribe medications, whereas the latter is unable to prescribe medications.

Dermatologists
Dermatologists are physicians who specialize in the treatment of disorders of the skin. They complete a 4-year residency, during which they become proficient in the identification and treatment of skin disorders, growths, and cancers. Dermatologists perform procedures to remove skin lesions, typically by freezing or cutting them off.

Physiatrists
Physiatrists are physicians who specialize in the treatment of musculoskeletal diseases and disorders that lead to a change or decline in function that may benefit from

treatments directed at rehabilitation. Physiatrists complete a 4-year residency. Their practice is commonly known as physical medicine and rehabilitation (PM&R). The physical medicine portion can be thought of as nonoperative orthopedics addressing pain and problems related to the musculoskeletal system. The rehabilitation aspect focuses on directing a team of therapists working to help a patient recover from a disorder that causes a significant change in function. Stroke, spinal cord injuries, traumatic brain injuries, and amputations are examples of such disorders. Additionally, physiatrists also perform electrodiagnostic studies or may perform spinal injections. Injections may address pain and decreased function secondary to disc herniations and spinal arthritis.

Radiologists

Radiologists are specialists who interpret diagnostic imaging studies. They complete a 4-year residency. Radiologists specialize in reading imaging studies. They are experts at reading CT scans, MRIs, radiographs (X-rays), and ultrasound studies. They may choose to do an interventional fellowship of 1 to 2 years to gain the additional skills necessary to use CT or X-rays to place catheters or to perform interventions to treat problems.

NEED TO KNOW

Board certification is the gold standard among physicians. This refers to the fact that the physician has completed a residency training program in his or her specialty as well as successfully passed an examination. This certification assures the patient of a certain level of standing. *Board eligible* denotes that the physician has completed the training but has not taken the test yet.

Figure Credits

7

Surgical Specialties

Objective

 ▸ Basic understanding of the different surgical specialists and subspecialists and familiarity with the procedures they perform

Definition

 ▸ *Surgeon:* A physician who makes his or her livelihood operating on the human body.

Hierarchy?

There is no hierarchy in medicine. The surgeon's recommendations do not overrule an internist's recommendations or vice versa. Physicians, including specialists, will generally treat patients from their point of view. For example, a cardiologist my recommend a medicine to lower cholesterol, but this may cause significant muscle pains in the patient as a side effect. The patient may then be seen by another specialist, who recommends discontinuing the medication. The patient will then need to determine what course of action to pursue. A similar situation may exist when deciding whether to have a surgery. Some decisions are obvious and do not require much debate or a second opinion, such as surgery to remove a cancerous tumor. Other surgeries may be elective. They have the potential to improve someone's medical status, but with any surgery there are risks involved. An elective surgery on the back may relieve the original debilitating back pain or result in scar tissue and an eventual increase in pain.

Second Opinion

It is best to get a second opinion regarding surgery if it is elective and the patient is not completely sure about the recommendation. Primary care physicians can also offer their input based on their experiences. Patients may worry that the original physician may be insulted by getting a second opinion, but most physicians are fairly comfortable with patients getting a second opinion. The patient may receive the same opinion, which may confirm what to do next. In medicine there may be different ways to treat the same problem. Therefore it is not insulting to get a second opinion. When a second opinion is attained, the patient will evaluate the input of the physicians and their treatment recommendations.

General Surgery

In medical school physicians in training will decide to follow a path of medicine or a surgical path following graduation from medical school. Similar to generalists and specialists in medicine, there are generalists and specialists in surgery. General surgery is a 5-year residency that is completed following medical school. General surgeons are trained to cover a broad area of diseases in most areas of the body that require surgery. They are also trained in the diagnosis and treatment of patients before, during, and after their surgeries. General surgeons will be trained in surgery involving the abdomen, breasts, and skin. Surgeries involving the brain, spine, thoracic region, and bones will typically be performed by specialists in those fields.

General surgeons will commonly remove infected appendixes and gallbladders. The removal of a gallbladder is known as a cholecystectomy. The gallbladder is removed secondary to infection or accumulation of stones in its wall or duct. The procedure to remove a gallbladder can be done either via an open approach or a laparoscopic one.

The open approach is the traditional method; it involves making a 3–5 inch incision in the abdomen to gain access to the organ. The recovery is typically longer, but the complication rate is lower than the laparoscopic approach. The laparoscopic approach uses a laparoscope, a device that permits viewing of the abdominal cavity. Three 1-inch or smaller incisions are used to permit the scopes to enter the abdominal cavity. Devices for viewing, a light source, and tools are used to remove the organ. The use of scopes to perform surgeries has become the standard of care for the majority of operations and procedures.

Cardiothoracic Surgery

Cardiothoracic surgeons are surgical specialists who perform surgery on the heart and repair adjacent vessels of the heart. Cardiothoracic surgeons complete a 5-year general surgery residency and an additional 3-year residency in cardiothoracic surgery. During their specialty training, they may focus on valve replacements, ventricular assist devices, and endoscopic techniques.

Transplantation Surgery

Transplant surgeons are surgical specialist who perform transplantation surgeries. They complete a 5-year general surgery residency followed by a 2-year fellowship in transplantation. They specialize in liver, kidney, and pancreas transplantations.

Transplant surgeons learn the operative techniques for organ procurement from deceased organ donors. They will also provide comprehensive care for transplant patients following surgery.

Otolaryngology

Otolaryngologists are surgeons who specialize in the treatment of the ears, nose, neck, and throat. Otolaryngologists complete a 5-year residency in otolaryngology. These surgeons are commonly referred to as ENTs (ear, nose, and throat). Otolaryngology specialists are trained in procedures related to the ear, nose, sinuses, larynx, head, and neck surgery. They commonly perform tonsillectomies, sinus surgeries, nasal septum surgeries such as septoplasties, and cancer resections involving the head and neck. They also commonly perform myringotomies, the placing of tubes in the ears for recurrent infections.

Plastic and Reconstructive Surgery

Plastic and reconstructive surgeons specialize in microsurgeries and reconstruction. They spend 6 years in a residency specializing in these skills. They are exposed to complex reconstructive surgeries involving the breast, head, neck, abdominal wall, and peripheral nerve procedures during their training. The plastics aspect of their field typically involves procedures done for cosmetic purposes, including breast augmentation and facial surgeries. The elective procedures are rarely covered by insurance, and patients will need to pay for these procedures from their own private funds. The reconstructive aspect of the field involves scar revision, cleft lip/palate repair, burned skin repair/revision, and reconstruction of the breasts following removal for cancer (mastectomy). Additional skills of plastic surgeons may involve reconstruction of injured nerves.

Neurosurgery

Neurosurgeons specialize in the treatment of the nervous system. They complete a 7-year residency. They specialize in the treatment and removal of brain/spinal tumors, hydrocephalus (swelling of the ventricles of the brain), and brain hemorrhages (bleeds). They may place a shunt in the brain to remove the increased fluid seen with hydrocephalus. They may also need to perform a craniotomy or drill holes in the skull to relieve pressure of the brain following a bleed or hemorrhage. Neurosurgeons are typically held in high esteem among medical professionals, given their extensive training, level of patient commitment, and call requirements.

Orthopedics

Orthopedic surgeons specialize in treatment of bone and musculoskeletal disorders. They complete a 5-year residency, during which they are taught all aspects of bone care, including traumatic fractures, tumors, degenerative arthritis, and sports-related injuries. They may specialize in joint replacement surgeries, including knee, hip, and shoulder replacements. Arthroscopic procedures (endoscopic procedures involving the joints) are commonly done in the knee, shoulder, and more recently the hip. The arthroscopic approach can repair torn ligaments and fix tears in the lining of the joints (debridements). Other orthopedic surgeons may choose to do a 1- to 2-year fellowship and further specialize in tumor resection, trauma care, or spine surgeries.

Fracture care also remains a keystone of orthopedic care. Orthopedic surgeons routinely perform surgeries to address fractures, including fractures that are not lined up, known as displaced fractures. The care of a displaced fracture may include placing the pieces in alignment (known as reduction) or utilizing hardware (screws and plates) to get the bone pieces or fragments to align together. Treatment for a nondisplaced fracture may involve placing a cast on the injured extremity. The goal is to reduce movement at the fracture site to promote healing of the bone.

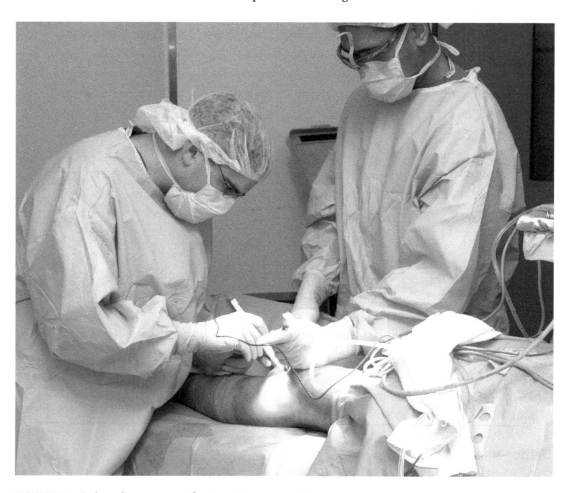

FIGURE 7.1   Orthopedic surgeons performing ACL reconstruction.

Figure Credit

8

Physician Office Visit

Objectives

- ▶ Basic understanding of the best way to prepare for an office visit
- ▶ Anatomy of an office visit
- ▶ Basic physical examination

Office Visits

The majority of health care administered in the United States is done not in a hospital but during an outpatient visit. According to the Centers for Disease Control and Prevention (CDC), there are 1.1 billion outpatient or office visits per year.[1] The CDC also notes that the average number of visits per person per year is four and the majority of visits, 53.2%, are to see a primary care physician. The most commonly diagnosed condition during these visits is arthritis and its related complications.

Options

Consumers have three main categories of doctors to choose from: a physician in academic practice, a physician who is employed by a health care system, and a physician who is in private practice. The differences are summarized in Table 8.1.

TABLE 8.1   DIFFERENT PHYSICIAN OPTIONS

Type	Pros	Cons
Academic	Complete visits	Long visits, multiple learners
Employed	Associated with health system	Pressures to perform
Private practice	Efficient and convenient visits	Financial incentives to see and do more

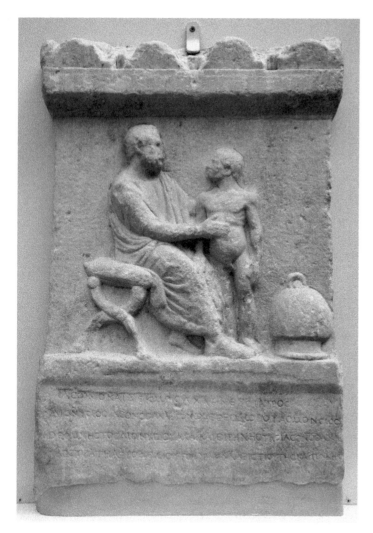

FIGURE 8.1 Marble relief of physician and patient, 2nd century AD.

Academic physicians work for a medical school and treat patients but also educate physicians in training, including medical students, interns, residents, and fellows. They are likely knowledgeable in terms of the latest treatments and evidence-based medicine. In addition, the medical school may offer clinical trials or novel treatments. Educating physicians in training may mean a patient is seen first by the resident or student, who will then present the patient's history and examination findings to the academic or attending physician. The attending physician will likely confirm important parts of the patient's history and may repeat certain portions of the physical examination. Visits tend to run on the long side, but are especially complete.

An employed physician is employed by a health care organization; the doctor is usually associated with other physicians and specialists in the health care network. Some health care systems may be associated with resident training programs but not typically medical students. The care has the advantage of being accessible to other providers within the health care system. The employed physician has pressure to see a certain number of patients and to do more for the health care system. The number of employed physicians has steadily increased over the past decade, while the number of private practice physicians has declined.

The private practice is another option for physicians. Private practice physicians may be affiliated with a hospital but are not employed by the hospital. Their practice is based on providing good, efficient care to patients. They may offer extended office hours with convenient accessibility, including parking. They are usually not associated with residents or other physicians in training. The private practice physician has a financial incentive to see patients and perform procedures or surgeries; for this reason, visits tend to be efficient.

Charges

The different physicians may bill the patient differently. The academic physician will submit a bill for professional charges, and any procedures that the physician performs in the academic medical center will be included in the professional charges. The employed physician will bill a professional component, and the health care system may submit a facility fee charge. The private practice physician will submit a single global fee that includes the professional component and facilities portion of the bill.

Establishing Care

When individuals have chosen a physician to provide care, they need to confirm that the physician accepts their insurance. Most providers will accept Medicare as well as private insurance. Finding physicians who accept Medicaid may be more challenging, especially private care providers. It is best to confirm that one's insurance product is accepted at a prospective physician's office before initiating care.

Appointment Scheduling

Patients' time to see a physician is typically scheduled, meaning they cannot simply show up to be seen. Unfortunately, it is not uncommon to wait in the office well beyond a scheduled appointment time. Some waits can be longer than 90 minutes, though most are less than 20 minutes. Why the delay in being seen later than the scheduled appointment time? One reason is the complexity of various problems. A patient may indicate a relatively simple problem at the time the appointment is made, but more time may be needed to better understand the problem. Also, very commonly patients will have more than one problem they wish to have addressed. This requires extra time, and the extra time can certainly build as the number of patients seen increases as the day goes on. Additionally, some patients arrive late to the office, which impedes the flow of the physician. If the 10:00 patient arrives 7 minutes late, then all subsequent patients will likely be delayed 7 minutes. The most recent factor is the advent of the electronic medical record, which adds additional time per patient to satisfy the multiple regulations that are required.

Appointment

When arriving at the office for an appointment, patients will notify the staff of their presence. It is important patients arrive with any radiograph studies or have them sent prior to their visit to the office. Staff are not allowed to identify patients by their last name because of the Health Insurance Portability and Accountability Act of 1996 (HIPAA). Therefore, the staff will call patients by their first name. Once called, the nursing staff will take patients to an examination room and obtain vital signs. These are standard measurements of temperature, heart rate, breathing rate, and blood pressure. Most offices will also obtain a height and weight.

A medical intake form, may have been sent prior to the appointment or can be filled out in the office while patients are waiting for the physician or care provider to enter the room. The medical intake form may also be done verbally, done when the patient gives the information to the nursing staff and it is entered electronically into your medical record. The staff will also ask patients the main reason for their visit, known as the "chief complaint." Certain care providers may stick to a "one-visit one-problem" approach. They will also review patients' past medical history, so it is best for patients to bring any previous medical records if they are unsure or cannot recall.

Allergies to medications will also be reviewed. There is a difference between an allergy and a sensitivity. A true allergy is a reaction, occasionally life threatening, to a medication. It can involve swelling of the lips, tongue, or throat or development of an itchy rash. Sensitivities to drugs are not severe reactions and may include nausea, diarrhea, sedation, and headache. Any current medications that patients are taking will also be reviewed. It is best to actually bring in the medication bottles to know exactly what a patient is taking; telling the nurse or physician one is taking a small pink pill does not help. Many medications look alike, and one generic producer may produce a different color and shaped pill than another manufacturer of the same medication.

Social history entails occupational or vocational review as well discussing alcohol or tobacco use. Family history may also be helpful in having a knowledge of certain diseases that run in the family. Knowing the health history of one's parents and siblings can be very beneficial. Lastly, patients may be asked to fill out a review of systems form. This will ask a number of questions related to the health or medical issues of the different systems of the body and may include the following: cardiac, pulmonary, neurologic, and orthopedic.

The physician, nurse practitioner, physician assistant, or other care provider will enter the room. It is important for patients to know that their scheduled appointment is 20 to 45 minutes for a new patient visit and 10 to 20 minutes for a follow-up visit. To get the most out of one's visit, it is best to be clear and concise with one's description of the problem. For example, when patients are asked how long they have had a certain pain, they should respond with a time duration answer—this is not the time to get into overly descriptive details of the day, such as the weather, what they were wearing the day the pain started, or how their normal routine was disrupted and the consequences that occurred. The correct answer takes seconds; while the convoluted approach wastes minutes and doesn't actually answer the original question. If the physician or care provider feels additional details are helpful, he or she will ask the circumstances further.

Physical Examination

The hallmark of any office visit is the physical examination, which doctors have been performing for greater than 2,000 years. The care provider will perform a physical examination. Depending on the problem, the examination may be comprehensive or focused. Comprehensive examinations will include examinations of multiple parts (organs) of the body, which may help in making a diagnosis. The focused examination will examine limited areas of the body that are parts related to the chief complaint.

Expectations

Following a medical office visit, patients should be provided with the following: diagnosis (cause of their disease, problem, or illness), answers to any questions, and a plan. Sometimes the diagnosis is not obvious and will require additional testing to determine; in these cases a differential (a number of possible) diagnosis should be discussed and reviewed. Patients (consumers) are paying for the services of the physician and should ask any questions they have in terms of the diagnosis, treatment plan, and follow-up care. Lastly, all visits should end with a plan or patients should be provided with a recommendation. The plan may include medications, therapies, or additional testing.

NEED TO KNOW

Best appointment times: There are certain appointment times when the wait time in the office can be significantly reduced. The first appointment of the day and the first appointment after lunch are prime spots to schedule to reduce one's wait time. The first patient has the advantage of not following any patient, so the provider will likely start on time. The wait times will likely increase as the day goes on. They will reset after the lunch break and build again as the afternoon progresses.

Reference

1. https://www.cdc.gov/nchs/pressroom/08newsreleases/visitstodoctor.htm

Figure Credit

9

The Pharmaceutical Industry

Objectives

- ▸ Basic understanding of the pharmaceutical industry
- ▸ Review of the role of the U.S. Food and Drug Administration
- ▸ Understanding of the past and current relationship between the pharmaceutical industry and physicians

Industry

The pharmaceutical industry develops, produces, and markets drugs or pharmaceuticals for use as medications to treat disease and ailments. The few companies that produce and market the drugs are large and control a very large share of the market. According to the World Health Organization (WHO), the 10 largest drugs companies control over one third of this market, several with sales of more than $10 billion a year and profit margins of about 30%. Six of these companies are based in the United States and four in Europe.

Development

Today medications undergo rigorous clinical trials and testing. This testing was implemented following the thalidomide tragedy in the 1960s. Thalidomide was a German-produced drug used to treat morning sickness during pregnancy. It was not extensively tested in pregnant animals, which was not the standard of the time. Unfortunately, the medication was associated with disastrous side effects to fetuses. Children were born either without or with severely deformed arms and legs. As a result of this tragedy, the World Medical Association set standards for clinical research.

Pharmaceutical companies are required to prove efficacy and safety of the drug in clinical trials before marketing them (see Table 9.1). This includes a four-step process, which is overseen by the *U.S. Food and Drug Administration*

TABLE 9.1   SUMMARY OF DRUG DEVELOPMENT TRIALS

Phase	Number of volunteers	Time	Goals	Percentage successful
1	20–100	Months	Safety	70%
2	100–500	Up to 2 years	Efficacy	33%
3	1,000–5,000	1–4 years	Efficacy and side effects	25%–30%
4	>5,000	Ongoing	Side effects	NA

(FDA). Phase 1 of testing includes drug tests in a small group of about 20 to 100 healthy volunteers. Testing is done to determine the safety of the drug. If the drug is not safe and causes significant side effects or cannot be tolerated, the testing will stop at this phase. If the drug is found to be safe for human consumption, testing will proceed. According to the FDA, about 70% of drugs move on to the next phase of testing.

The second phase of testing will involve 100 to 500 volunteer patients in controlled trials. The purpose of the second phase is to determine the efficacy (whether the medicine is effective) in treating the disease as well as look at side effects. If found in controlled trials to be effective, the drug moves on to the next phase. The FDA estimates that 33% of medications will make it to the third phase of testing.

The third phase includes 1,000 to 5,000 patients who take the drug and are monitored to confirm effectiveness and also to identify any side effects. This trial will have some of the volunteers take the new medication and others take a placebo (compound or intervention with no active drug effects). This is done to compare the side effects of the medication with the placebo. The FDA estimates that 25% to 30% of medications pass this phase.

During the fourth and final phase, trials are carried out once the drug has been approved by the FDA during the post market safety monitoring. In summary, for every 100 drugs produced, 70 will make it to phase 2, 23 will make it to phase 3, and 6 will be approved by the FDA after a period of testing of ranging from 2 to 7 years.

Research

Companies currently spend one third of all sales revenue on marketing their products, roughly twice what they spend on research and development. As a result of this pressure to maintain sales, there is now, in WHO's words, "an inherent conflict of interest between the legitimate business goals of manufacturers and the social, medical and economic needs of providers and the public to select and use drugs in the most rational way."[1]

This is particularly true when drugs companies are the main source of information as to which products are most effective. The industry expanded rapidly in the 1960s, benefiting from new discoveries, and there were attempts to try to limit the financial links between drug companies and physicians. No legislation was enacted at that time. Without limits, the industry created and effectively used sales representatives to influence physician prescribing.

Marketing

The pharmaceutical industry has historically utilized sales representatives, also known as drug reps, to influence physicians' prescribing patterns. The drug reps are typically young, energetic, and attractive. They will visit physicians in their office to tell them about new medications or to update them on current medications. Their goal is to increase the sale of their medication. Drug reps are typically assigned a geographic area and certain medication brands produced by the pharmaceutical company. The company will track how well the rep is doing based on sales of that drug in that particular region.

In order to get a busy physician's attention, the rep would provide a catered lunch for the entire office, in exchange for a few minutes of the physician's time. During this time the rep would educate the physician on the medication and any recent studies to show the medication's superiority over other treatments. In addition, the rep would give the office pens, notepads, and other items emblazed with the medication's name to further remind the doctor and his or her staff of the medication. In the past, in certain circumstances drug reps would take physicians on trips or a day of golfing to develop a better relationship with the physician. One drug rep, Gwen Olsen, has written a book titled *Confessions of an Rx Drug Pusher*, detailing her 15 years as a pharmaceutical representative and her associated experiences.

Out of concern over the influence drug reps have on physician prescribing patterns, academic medical centers have restricted or limited the access of drug reps. The pharmaceutical industry then went to another approach. It enlisted the assistance of physicians to get the word out to other physicians.

The pharmaceutical companies would sponsor a dinner, typically at a very nice restaurant, and have a physician serve as a lecturer at the dinner. The physician would talk about the merits of a particular medication the company was sponsoring and in exchange receive an honorarium (payment) for the lecture. This approach was effective. "An internal study done by Merck & Co. several years ago calculated the 'return on investment' from doctor-led discussion groups was almost double the return on meetings led by the company's own sales force. According to the document, doctors who attended a lecture by another doctor wrote an additional $623.55 worth of prescriptions for the painkiller Vioxx over a 12-month period compared with doctors who didn't attend. That compared to an increase of only $165.87 in Vioxx prescriptions by doctors who attended a meeting with a salesperson."[2]

On the national level, legislation addressing these concerns has been enacted. The Physician Payments Sunshine Act created the Open Payments Program, administered by the Centers for Medicare & Medicaid Services. The program is designed to create greater transparency around the financial relationships between the pharmaceutical industry, physicians, and teaching hospitals. The Sunshine Act began on August 1, 2013, and requires certain pharmaceutical and device manufacturers to report payments or other transfers of value given to U.S. physicians and teaching hospitals. Reports are made yearly, and the information is accessible to the public on the web. Manufacturers must report payments or transfer of value for the following: funding for research, travel, honoraria, speaking fees, and meals.

The website link of this CMS site is listed at the end of this chapter.

Marketing dollars have now been shifted away from drug reps and physicians and spent on advertising directly to the consumers or patients. The aim of this direct-to-consumer advertising is for patients to learn of medications and ask for them by name at their physician's office. There has been a significant increase in drug advertisements on television. The United States is one of the few countries that still permit pharmaceutical advertising on television. The ads, much like other ads, target a certain demographic group during a particular program. Evening news ads will target the elderly with medications for chronic pain and other problems, while sporting events may advertise erectile dysfunction medication directed at males. The idea is to influence consumers or patients, who will ask for the medication by name, putting pressure on their treating physician to prescribe the medication.

There have been some negative consequences with limiting pharmaceutical samples in physician offices. One concern was that the samples were trialed to determine if they could help a patient. For example, patches for pain were given in a limited supply, perhaps three to a patient to trial them, and if they were effective then a prescription could be filled. Now without samples, the patient will instead get a prescription filled, and since certain patches come in a box of 30, some pharmacists are reluctant to give out only 3—meaning the patient needs to get an entire box, which is expensive and may not be effective. Also, samples could be given to try to supplement medication supply with the costs of getting the prescriptions filled. Samples of a few weeks would reduce the financial burden of having to pay for the medications. Lastly, physicians may not be informed as to new treatments and medications that are available and may hear about them first from a patient during a visit.

It is important for consumers to keep in mind the influence pharmaceutical companies can have over them and physicians in terms of advertising. When asking a physician about a medication, a good approach is to mention the medication and ask the physician of his or her experiences with the medication. Additionally, if one's doctor is insistent on prescribing a certain medication, a good question to ask is whether there is a less expensive alternative. In the world of medications, newer is not always necessarily better. Aspirin has been around for greater than a century and is a very effective treatment for reducing the risk of both heart attack and stroke. Newer and more expensive medications are available but may not improve outcomes much, if any—and at a substantially higher cost.

Given the costs of medications, they should be prescribed if they work and continue to work. Medications should not be taken if they are supposed to work and no change is noted in the patient. For example, if a patient starts a new medication to lower blood pressure and no effect is noted, the medication should be discontinued and another class of medication tried.

NEED TO KNOW

The FDA, which was created in 1906 by an act of the U.S. Congress, regulates the modern pharmaceutical industry. The agency is also a scientific and public health agency with oversight for the safety of most food products, radiation-emitting consumer products, cosmetics, and animal feed.[3]

References

1. http://www.who.int/medicines/areas/quality_safety/quality_assurance/norms_standards/en/
2. Hensley, S., & Martinez, B. (2005, July 15). To sell their drugs, companies increasingly rely on doctors: For $750 and up, physicians tell peers about products; talks called educational. *The Wall Street Journal.* Retrieved from https://www.wsj.com/articles/SB112138815452186385
3. Pharmaceutical industry. (2008). *International Encyclopedia of the Social Sciences.* Retrieved from http://www.encyclopedia.com
4. https://www.fda.gov/forpatients/approvals/drugs/ucm405622.htm

Resources

Centers for Medicare & Medicaid Services—Open Payments is a national disclosure program that promotes a transparent and accountable health care system by making the financial relationships between applicable manufacturers (pharmaceuticals) and medical organizations and health care providers available to the public: https://www.cms.gov/openpayments/

Gwen Olsen-Site founded by Gwen Olsen former pharmaceutical rep, devoted to educating the public in regards to medications and fostered improved outcomes: http://gwenolsen.com/

Food and Drug Administration—Website that reviews the process of medication approval from the FDA, serves to expand the consumers knowledge of getting the medication to the public: https://www.fda.gov/forpatients/approvals/drugs/ucm405622.htm

World Health Organization—Home site of the organization devoted to improving global health: http://www.who.int/en/

Prescriptions and Medications

Prescription

A prescription is a written order or message from a doctor to a pharmacist, therapist, or medical supplier directing the individual to dispense or initiate the use of a medicine, therapy, or medical equipment. Historically, prescriptions have been written on prescription paper. More recently, the federal government has encouraged prescribers to send the prescriptions electronically. There are inherent advantages to using e-prescribing. After the initial input, prescriptions are more convenient to renew. Another significant advantage is legibility; handwritten prescriptions can sometimes be very hard to read or decipher, and many medications have similar-looking names. Unfortunately, this has resulted in errors such as filling the wrong prescriptions and patient morbidity and mortality. For example, amiodarone is a medication for heart arrhythmias, while amantadine is used to treat the flu or abnormal movements associated with Parkinson's disease. They are both 10 letters long and if not clearly written could be mistaken for each other, with potentially devastating complications. Prescriptions may also be phoned into the pharmacy by physicians or their office staff.

Most prescriptions were traditionally written on a prescription paper. This paper is usually printed and contains the physician's name, business address, and additional contact information. Some prescriptions are printed on tamper-proof paper so they cannot be easily altered. In reality, the prescription can be written on a napkin, as long as it contains the following: physician's name and address, the patient's name and date of birth, date of the prescription, and the prescription information. This information includes the name of the

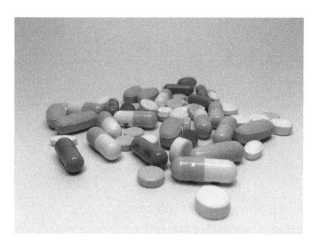

FIGURE 10.1   Medications.

medication and dosage (usually in milligrams, or mg), how many to dispense, how to take them— by mouth, injection, or topically (applied to the skin)—how often to take them, and how many refills are allowed.

Controlled Substances Act

The Controlled Substances Act is the statute prescribing U.S. federal drug policy and under which the manufacture, importation, possession, use, and distribution of certain substances is regulated. It was passed by the 91st U.S. Congress as Title II of the Comprehensive Drug Abuse Prevention and Control Act of 1970 and signed into law by President Richard Nixon.[1]

This legislation created five schedules (classifications), based on the addictive potential of the medication. Two federal agencies, the Drug Enforcement Administration (DEA) and the FDA, determine which substances are added to or removed from the various schedules. The FDA, which was created in 1906 by an act of Congress, regulates the modern pharmaceutical industry.[2] The Controlled Substance Staff is located within the FDA's Center for Drug Evaluation and Research. The Controlled Substance Staff evaluates all drugs that have an effect on the central nervous system. Such drugs may have a stimulant, depressant, or hallucinogenic effect. The drug classes that are commonly tested include ones classified as opioids, stimulants, hallucinogens, benzodiazepines, barbiturates, cannabinoids, and anabolic steroids. The Controlled Substance Staff assesses the actual abuse data to determine whether a drug under review requires abuse potential studies and scheduling. The Controlled Substance Staff also conveys abuse-related messages. The DEA was created by Nixon through an executive order in July 1973 in order to establish a single unified command to combat "an all-out global war on the drug menace."[3] The DEA enforces the laws of regulation.

Drug Schedules

Drugs, substances, and certain chemicals used to make drugs are classified into five distinct categories, or schedules, depending on the drug's acceptable medical use and the drug's abuse or dependency potential. The abuse rate is a determinate factor in the scheduling of the drug. The schedules are summarized in Table 10.1.

Schedule I drugs, substances, or chemicals are defined as drugs with no currently accepted medical use and a high potential for abuse. They are believed to be the most

TABLE 10.1   SUMMARY OF CONTROLLED SUBSTANCE CATEGORIES

Category	Addiction Potential	Examples	Rx
I	Extremely high	Heroin, LSD, marijuana, and ecstasy	None
II	Very high	Hydrocodone, cocaine, Adderall, methadone, Dilaudid, Demerol, OxyContin, fentanyl, and Ritalin	30-day supply
III	Moderate	T3(Tylenol with codeine), ketamine, anabolic steroids, and testosterone	30-day (or more) refills
IV	Reduced	Xanax, Soma, Valium, Ativan, Talwin, Ambien, and tramadol	30-day (or more) refills
V	Low	Robitussin AC, Lomotil, Lyrica, and Parepectolin	30-day (or more) refills

dangerous drugs of all the drug schedules, with potentially severe psychological or physical dependence. Some examples of Schedule I drugs are heroin, LSD, marijuana, and ecstasy.

It is interesting to note that marijuana is a Schedule I drug but is legal in certain states for recreational and/or medical use. In August 2016 the DEA reaffirmed its stance on marijuana being a Schedule I drug. Certain states were hoping for a drop to Schedule II, but the DEA did permit expanded research into the medical effects of marijuana. The federal law supersedes the state laws. However, the DEA has not taken action against the states that have legalized marijuana for medical or recreational use. The Justice Department has reserved its right to challenge state laws if public health problems occur in the states that have legalized marijuana.

Schedule II drugs are defined as drugs with a very high potential for abuse, with use potentially leading to severe psychological or physical dependence. These drugs are also considered potentially dangerous but have been shown to have medical value. Some examples of Schedule II drugs are Adderall, cocaine, Demerol, Dilaudid, Lortab, methadone, OxyContin, Percocet, Ritalin, and Vicodin. Despite the fact that it is unlawful to possess or take a controlled Schedule II substance without a prescription, the medications are shared, stolen, diverted, and sold. Any patient who is under a physician's care for Substance II medications is required to be seen by the physician every 90 days. The prescriptions have historically been limited to a 30-day supply with no refills, although this regulation may be changing.

Some medications to treat attention-deficit/hyperactivity disorder (ADHD) and attention-deficit disorder (ADD) fall into this category. The medications Ritalin and Adderall are controlled Schedule II substances, and for this reason it is illegal to share, buy, or borrow these medications. They work to stimulate the attention centers of the brain in individuals with ADD and ADHD, but have not been shown to improve intelligence, the ability to study, or the ability to do better on tests in subjects without ADD or ADHD. Nonetheless, they are subject to resale on campuses throughout the country for the false belief they will aid intellectual pursuits.

Schedule III drugs exhibit a moderate to low potential for physical and psychological dependence. Codeine is a medication that can be habit forming and serves as the basis for Schedule III drugs. The following are examples of Schedule III drugs: products containing less than 90 milligrams of codeine per dosage unit such as Tylenol with codeine, ketamine, anabolic steroids, and testosterone. Schedule III drugs can be written for a greater than 30-day supply and are refillable. In addition, the prescription can be called into a pharmacy.

Schedule IV drugs have a low potential for abuse and low risk of dependence. Some examples of Schedule IV drugs are Xanax, Soma, Valium, Ativan, Talwin, Ambien, and tramadol. Use of this schedule of medications should not be taken lightly; they can still present problems with physical dependence and withdrawal, particularly Xanax and Valium. The use and addictive potential of tramadol (brand name Ultram) also appears to be on the rise.

Schedule V drugs are drugs that have lower potential for abuse than Schedule IV and consist of preparations containing limited quantities of certain narcotics. Schedule V drugs are generally used for antidiarrheal, antitussive, and analgesic purposes. Some examples of Schedule V drugs are cough preparations with less than 200 milligrams of codeine or per 100 milliliters such as Robitussin AC, Lomotil, Lyrica, and Parepectolin.

Addiction

Abuse as defined by the Controlled Substance Staff is the intentional nontherapeutic use of a drug, even once, to achieve a desired psychological or physiological effect. The Controlled Substance Staff defines drug addiction as a cluster of behavioral, cognitive, and physiological phenomena that may include a strong desire to take the drug, difficulties in controlling drug use (e.g., continuing drug use despite harmful consequences, giving a higher priority to drug use than any other activities and obligations), and possible tolerance or physical dependence.

Addiction is a growing problem in America currently, with federal and state programs trying to address this problem. Why is there such a problem? Medications used for pain (narcotics) have no ceiling effect, which means they can continue to be raised as the patient develops tolerance. Tolerance is developed as the liver adapts to metabolizing the medication. In addition, there can be receptor changes at the level of the central nervous system, where the drugs interact, as well as pleasurable feelings in certain centers of the brain with their use.

An additional factor regarding addiction is the prescribing of narcotic medications for chronic nonmalignant (noncancerous) pain. These will help initially, but then as the patient develops tolerance the dosage will need to be increased. After it is increased, the pain will be improved for a time, but then the dosage will need to be increased; the cycle continues until a point that the prescribing physician may not feel comfortable increasing further. Narcotics are not medications that can be abruptly stopped, as this will lead to withdrawal. Withdrawal is not life threatening but is an awful experience that some patients have described as the worst feeling of their lives. That is a significant component to the reason that getting patients off the medication can be so difficult. In order to get off the addictive medication, a patient must want to get off the medication, and a slow taper of the medication with education regarding withdrawal is a necessary part of the plan.

Medications in Pregnancy

In addition to their possible addiction potential, medications are also classified according to their risks to the fetus if taken during pregnancy. The drugs are classified in categories starting with A, summarized in Table 10.2. Medications in the class have had adequate and well-controlled studies that have shown no risk to the fetus in the first semester (the time that a fetus is the most vulnerable to complications associated with cell differentiation).

Category B medications are without well-controlled studies in pregnant women, while animal studies have not shown there to be a risk to the fetus. *Category C* medications have been shown in animal studies to have an adverse effect on the developing fetus; there are no adequate human studies. The risk–benefit ratio must be carefully looked at when deciding to take Category C medications during pregnancy. *Category D* medications have evidence of human fetal risk based on adverse reaction data. *Category X* medications have been shown in both animal and human studies to be associated with fetal abnormalities. Lastly, *Category N* is the classification in which the FDA has not studied the drug.

TABLE 10.2   CLASSIFICATIONS OF MEDICINES DURING PREGNANCY

Category	Human studies	Animal studies
A	No risk	No risk
B	No studies	No risk
C	No studies	Adverse effects
D	Adverse reactions	Adverse effects
X	Fetal abnormalities	Fetal abnormalities
N	No studies	No studies

Placebo

Placebo can be a pill, injection, or procedure that has no proven medical benefit but results in a positive or beneficial health outcome. It is the result of individuals' anticipation that the treatment or medication will help them. There are a few factors that can influence the outcome of a placebo: one is the physician's interaction with patient, and another is related to the intrinsic beliefs of the patient. Placebo effect is on pain response. Experiments in the 1950s involved giving one group of patients a salt tablet and the other group morphine for pain control following an operation. The effectiveness of the placebo response is usually around 30%.

Generic Medication

Generic medications are a way to substantially reduce the costs associated with prescriptions. Generic medications are bioequivalent to a brand name drug. They are produced after the patent on the medication has expired. According to the FDA, the patent length is currently 20 years from the date on which the application for the patent was filed in the United States. The generics are produced in the same dosage amount and quality as the brand medication. They are sold at discounted prices, since there is likely no need for marketing and advertising costs associated with the drug.

Copay Structure

Most insurance products offer a tier system regarding payment for medications. A three-tier system is the most common. Tier 1 medications include generic medications and have the lowest copay or may not require a copay at all. Tier 2 medications are preferred brand name medications associated with a higher copay amount. Tier 3 medications are nonpreferred medications and require the highest copay amount. The copay amounts have increased over the past few years. Different insurance carriers offer different preferred formularies. If you have a choice in selecting your insurance plan, knowing their formulary and matching it to your medication needs may be financially beneficial.

Over-the-Counter Medications

Over-the-counter (OTC) medications are sold directly to the consumer. No prescription is necessary to obtain the medication. Anti-inflammatory medicines for arthritis pain are the most commonly used OTC medications. OTC medications can have significant side effects and can certainly interact with prescription medications one may be taking. It is important to let your physician know what medications you are taking, including OTC meds. No medication is completely free of side effects.

References

1. Pub.L. 91–513, 84 Stat. 1236, enacted October 27, 1970, codified at 21 U.S.C. § 801 et. Seq.
2. Pharmaceutical industry. (2008). *International Encyclopedia of the Social Sciences.* Retrieved from http://www.encyclopedia.com
3. Drug Enforcement Administration. (n.d.). DEA history. Retrieved from http://www.dea.gov/about/history.shtml.

Resource

Food and Drug Administration—Link is to a manual detailing basic concepts regarding controlled substances and addiction, the definition section of the manual does a great job of comparing and defining the various terms associated with addiction: https://www.fda.gov/downloads/AboutFDA/ReportsManuals-Forms/StaffPoliciesandProcedur es/ucm073580.pdf

Figure Credit

Fig. 10.1: Copyright © NIAID (CC by 2.0) at https://commons.wikimedia.org/wiki/File:Assorted_Medications_(33931804863).jpg.

Diagnostic Laboratory Tests

11

Objective

▶ Basic understanding of the different diagnostic laboratory tests that are ordered in medicine and how they assist in treatments

Diagnosis

Diagnosis is the medical term used to define the determining cause of one's medical symptoms. It involves the process of coming to the conclusion of the underlying cause of one's problems based on the patient's history, examination, and review of laboratory data. It is commonly taught in medical school that the history and physical examination should provide the diagnosis about 75% of the time. Diagnostic tests can be helpful to confirm the diagnosis, follow the clinical status of the patient and disease process, and narrow the diagnosis if it is uncertain.

Diagnostic tests are medical procedures that can include laboratory tests, imaging tests, and other specialized tests. Laboratory tests are medical procedures that involve testing samples of blood, urine, or other tissues or substances in the body. Imaging tests help evaluate the anatomy of the body. Specialized tests are used to evaluate the functioning or physiology of the body and can include EKGs, sleep studies, pulmonary function tests, and EEGs.

Complete Blood Count

Common blood tests involve analysis of blood cells, electrolytes, and the function of certain organs. *Complete blood count* (*CBC*) is the test that looks at the population of blood cells in the body. Blood cells are produced by the marrow. Marrow is found in the middle or hollow portion of the long bones of our body. The marrow produces three main lines of cells: white cells, red cells, and platelets.

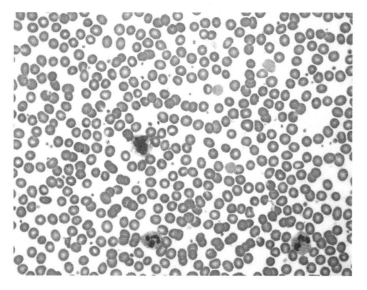

FIGURE 11.1   Normal blood smear showing red and white blood cells.

The three lines of cells perform different functions for the body. White blood cells, also known as leukocytes, are cells of the immune system and are important for fighting infections. The infections are caused by foreign invaders; bacteria, viruses, or fungi that can cause illness. Red blood cells are also known as erythrocytes, function to carry oxygen to the various organs of the body. Oxygen is used as a fuel for cell functions. Platelets are the other component of the blood; they function to prevent and stop bleeding by clumping together.

A CBC is ordered to evaluate the status of the three main cell lines. The blood test can give information about potential problems. There are normal ranges and parameters for the different cell lines. If the white blood cell (WBC) count is elevated, this may suggest an infection or leukemia. The WBCs can be followed to ensure the body or medications are adequately addressing the infection. Low WBCs can be caused by a viral infection, seen with chemotherapy, a toxic reaction, or a problem with the bone marrow that produces the cells.

The WBCs are able to be differentiated further into five subtypes—neutrophils, eosinophils, basophils, monocytes, and lymphocytes—based on their specific function. When the CBC is ordered, the ordering physician may request a manual differential, which entails having someone review the blood sample under a microscope to analyze and count the different subtypes of WBCs.

Neutrophils focus on fighting infections, particularly bacterial and fungal. Lymphocytes may be further differentiated into T and B cells. T cells aid in recognizing infections and serve to activate other immune cells. While B cells produce antibodies, which target invading germs. Monocytes are cells that may turn into macrophages. These cells can then engulf and eliminate infectious organisms, particularly bacteria. Eosinophils are important in fighting parasitic infections and are also involved with allergic responses. Lastly, basophils are important in the allergy cascade.

The red blood cell (RBC) count gives information about the oxygen-carrying capacity in the blood. The lab will describe one's RBC capacity in terms of hematocrit and hemoglobin. The hematocrit is the volume of red blood cells in your body, and it measures the ratio of RBCs in your blood. Hemoglobin is the iron-containing protein molecule in red blood cells that carries oxygen. Low RBC counts are known as anemia and can be caused by blood loss (bleeding) or lack of adequate iron in the body. The RBCs can be followed to assess response to treatment.

The platelets are also measured. Low platelet counts are known as thrombocytopenia and may be caused by a lack of production or an increase in destruction. Potential causes of low-production thrombocytopenia include viruses, leukemias, and chemotherapy. Increased destruction of platelets may be caused by pregnancy or autoimmune diseases.

Electrolytes

Electrolytes are electrically charged ions that regulate our nerve and muscle function and play a role in our body's pH. The pH system describes how acidic or alkaline a solution is, acidic solutions have a lower pH and alkaline solutions have a higher pH. The electrolytes exert control over ion channels in the nerves and muscles by generating electricity, contracting muscles, and affecting fluid concentrations within the body. The major electrolytes found within the body include: sodium, potassium, calcium, magnesium, phosphate, and chloride. The concentration of electrolytes in the body is dependent on their intake, as they cannot be produced by the body. Once in the body, they are regulated by hormones, mainly produced by the kidneys and adrenal glands. Sensors located within the kidneys monitor the specific concentrations of electrolytes. The kidneys will then determine when to filter and when to excrete the various electrolytes.

Since they play an important role in nerve and muscle activities, an imbalance of electrolytes can signal problems. The lab test that is ordered to evaluate the electrolytes involves taking a small sample of blood. It is commonly referred to as the basic metabolic panel or the Chem 8, as it usually contains eight tests. The electrolytes sodium, potassium, chloride, carbon dioxide (bicarbonate), and calcium account for five tests. Glucose, blood urea nitrogen, and creatinine make up the remaining three components. Together they will help provide the concentrations of the electrolytes in the body. Knowing the concentration can give important information as to the status of the kidneys and respiratory system.

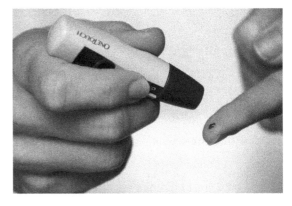

Blood Glucose

A blood glucose test is a laboratory test that takes a small sample of blood to measure the concentration of glucose in the blood. Glucose is a sugar, and its concentrations are regulated by hormones produced by the pancreas. The hormone that lowers the blood glucose level is insulin. The hormone that raises the blood glucose level is glucagon. The levels of glucose

FIGURE 11.2   Blood Glucose Testing.

are tested to determine if one has diabetes mellitus, which would be suggested by an elevated fasting blood glucose level. The level of glucose is expected to rise after eating a meal, and in response the body releases insulin to lower the level of glucose in the bloodstream. With diabetes, the body is unable to produce enough insulin or the body has developed a degree of resistance to insulin, and the blood glucose levels remain high. Elevated blood glucose levels over time can lead to destruction of nerves and injury to very small blood vessels. These issues can lead to blindness; loss of sensation in the feet, hands, and legs; and kidney damage. Medications can help improve blood glucose levels. Diabetics may need to monitor their levels to ensure some degree of blood glucose control with treatments.

Liver Function Tests

Liver function tests are blood tests that specifically evaluate the components of enzymes and proteins that are associated with proper liver functioning. The liver is the largest internal organ of the body (second overall to the skin). It serves many functions within the body. Liver function tests will look at each of the specific functions of the liver.

The liver is responsible for detoxification. It contains a number of enzymes that are responsible for converting drugs, alcohol, and toxins into harmless products that the body eliminates with bile in the intestines or excretes via the kidneys. Nutrients are also processed in the liver after they are digested. The liver will also produce bile, which is stored in the gallbladder and used to help break down fats and remove waste from the body. The liver also produces proteins necessary for blood clotting.

The liver is also important for storage of fat-soluble vitamins, as well as converting glucose into glycogen for storage. Its role in storing glucose also allows it to play a role

TABLE 11.1   SUMMARY AND FUNCTION OF LIVER FUNCTION TESTS

Name	Function
ALT	Liver enzyme test used in detoxifying; may suggest hepatocellular damage
AST	Liver enzyme test used in detoxifying; may suggest hepatocellular damage
Alk Phos	May indicate a problem with gallbladder or digestive tract
GGT	Liver enzyme test used in detoxifying and marker of alcohol disease
Protein	Measure of protein storing and processing function
Albumin	Measure of synthetic protein abilities
Prothrombin	Protein reflective of blood clotting function
Total bilirubin	Measurement of the ability to appropriately secrete
Direct bilirubin	Measurement of the ability to appropriately secrete

in blood sugar regulation. The specific lab tests involved with liver function tests and their role in the function of the liver are outlined in Table 11.1.

Kidney Function Tests

Kidney function tests are blood tests that are ordered to evaluate the functional status of the kidneys. These two organs are located in the retro (behind) peritoneal (abdominal cavity) region, one on either side. The kidneys are responsible for filtering and excreting waste products from the blood. They also assist in maintaining electrolyte balance and red blood cell production. In addition, they assist with red blood cell production and blood pressure regulation by means of hormone secretions. The labs of interest are the blood urea nitrogen, creatinine, and glomerular filtration rate. When the kidneys become impaired they are not able to actively secrete urea and creatinine out of the body and their levels become elevated. The glomerular filtration rate measures the ability of the kidney to filter; a normal level is greater than 60. A level lower than 60 but greater than 15 indicates kidney or renal impairment. Renal failure is a level that is lower than 15. The labs indicate that there is a problem with the kidney but do not specifically diagnose the problem, since the problem can be related to the blood flow before it enters the kidney (pre-renal), problem of the kidney itself (renal), or a problem in the ureters or bladder (post-renal) cause. Additional testing may be needed to further locate the exact cause.

NEED TO KNOW

Mononucleosis is also known as the "kissing disease." It is caused by the Epstein–Barr virus. The virus can be spread in saliva; hence the name kissing disease. It is very common among teenagers and college students. The diagnosis can be made on clinical grounds and confirmed with blood work. The CBC will show an elevated WBC with a differential showing elevated levels of monocytes and reduced neutrophils. The only treatment for mono is rest and supportive care for the associated symptoms. Recovery can take from 4 to 6 weeks or longer. During this time symptoms will include fatigue, muscle aches, sore throat, and swollen lymph nodes. The monocytes will collect in the spleen, so splenic enlargement may also occur. It is especially important to evaluate for splenic enlargement in active or athletic patients, as they are not allowed to return to contact sports until the spleen size has normalized. The enlarged spleen is susceptible to rupture, particularly from trauma.

Resource

National Institute of Diabetes and Digestive and Kidney Diseases—Webpage outlines basics of kidney diseases and how to monitor/treat the various conditions: https://www.niddk.nih.gov/health-information/health-communication-programs/nkdep/learn/causes-kidney-disease/testing/understand-gfr/Pages/understand-gfr.aspx

Figure Credits

12

Diagnostic Imaging Tests

Objective

▸ Basic understanding of the different diagnostic imaging tests that are ordered in medicine and how they assist with diagnosis and treatments

Diagnosis

Diagnosis is the medical term used to define the determining cause of one's medical symptoms. It involves the process of coming to the conclusion of the underlying cause of one's problems based on the patient's history, examination, and review of laboratory data. It is commonly taught in medical school that the history and physical examination should provide the diagnosis about 75% of the time. Diagnostic tests can be helpful to confirm the diagnosis, follow the clinical status of the patient and disease process, and narrow the diagnosis if it is uncertain.

Diagnostic tests are medical procedures that can include laboratory tests, imaging tests, and other specialized tests. Imaging tests help evaluate the anatomy of the body.

Radiograph

A radiograph is a photographic image produced by the action of an electromagnetic wave of high energy, known as an X-ray. To obtain an X-ray or radiograph, the patient is positioned between the X-ray source and a detector (film). The beam of energy passes through the body. When the X-ray passes through the different parts of the body, each part will absorb the X-rays in different amounts. The density of the tissue will determine how much radiation is absorbed. Bones—which are dense and made of calcium—will absorb more of the X-rays than softer tissues such as organs, muscles, and fat. The denser structures will appear white, and softer structures will range from gray to black.

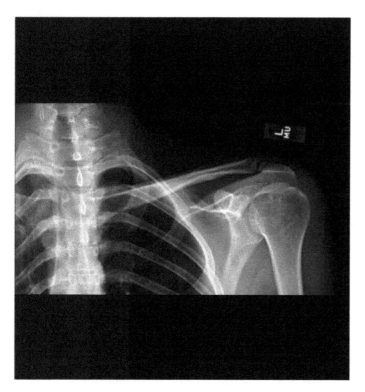

FIGURE 12.1 X-ray of the clavicle (collar bone).

X-rays are used primarily in patients to evaluate the status of a bone, evaluate the condition of the lungs, and determine the presence of a foreign body. When evaluating the status of a bone or bones, the X-ray can reveal if a bone is fractured. It can determine if the fracture is compound (multiple pieces) or displaced (edges of the fractures are not close to each other). Knowing this information assists in treatment; nondisplaced fractures can be splinted or casted, while displaced fractures will need to be reduced or surgically repaired. The X-rays can also show if the fracture and bone are healing appropriately. New bone growth at a fracture site is known as callus; serial radiographs can be taken to show the various stages of healing and callus formation.

Radiographs can also assist in gaining information about various processes in the lung. They can show lung changes that occur with COPD; they also may show the presence of a lung tumor or cancer. In addition, X-rays can reveal pneumonia (infection of the lung) and the presence of heart congestion and fluid buildup in the lungs. Lastly, they can reveal the presence of a pneumothorax (collapsed lung), which is a concern with trauma to the chest.

Additionally, radiographs can show the presence of a foreign body. This may assist in treating a young nonverbal child who may have swallowed a battery or other foreign object. The X-ray can also assist in evaluating a laceration of the extremity with glass to ensure a piece of glass is not embedded under the skin to avoid having a medical professional suture the laceration with the glass within the wound site.

CT Scan

Computerized axial tomography also knows as a CT or CAT scan, uses radiation to obtain a more detailed view of the body than regular radiographs. It was invented by an engineer, Godfrey Hounsfield, who was awarded the Noble Peace Prize in Medicine and was promoted by a neuroradiologist, James Ambrose, who demonstrated its wide clinical significance.[1] While the radiograph sends out a single X-ray, whereas the CAT scan sends out several beams from different angles. The different images are then

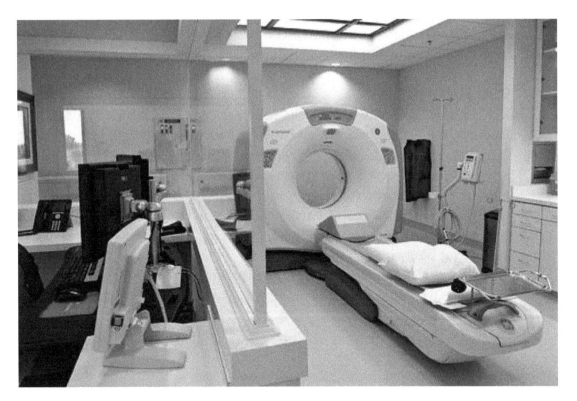

FIGURE 12.2 MRI scanner in which the patient is moved into the scanner.

processed by a computer, which creates axial (cross-sectional) images of the body. This allows for greater detail of images from within the body to be analyzed. The images are typically interpreted by a radiologist. The CAT scan does use radiation to obtain the images.

The CAT scanner, invented by Hounsfield, was originally designed to take pictures of the brain. It has been advanced and is now used to take images throughout the body. Advantages of the CAT scan include speed in obtaining images and the view of structures within the body. It is for this reason that the CAT scan is used in the initial evaluation of stroke patients who present to the hospital. The CAT scan can show if the suspected stroke is caused by a bleed or related to ischemia (lack of blood flow). Knowing this can direct the initial treatment of the stoke patient and lead to an improved outcome.

CAT scan imaging can be done preoperatively to evaluate a mass or tumor that can assist the surgeon in removal as well as guide an interventional radiologist in obtaining a biopsy of an organ or tissue sample. The CAT scan is particularly useful in the evaluation of bone and detecting the presence of a nondisplaced fracture, which may not show on a standard X-ray. The scans can also be used to follow an aortic abdominal aneurysm, assessing for enlargements. CAT scans are also used by radiation oncologist to precisely pinpoint the tumor for treatment with a beam of radiation.

Bone Scan

A bone scan is a nuclear imaging test that helps diagnose and track several types of bone problems. The testing procedure involves injecting a small amount of radioactive dye in the arm. X-ray pictures of the body are then taken. The X-rays can be of the entire body or a specific area of concern. Depending on the indication of the test, additional X-rays may be taken again after a period of 2 to 4 four hours. The uptake of the dye will be increased in "hot spots." Problems such as infections, fractures (not apparent on regular X-rays), and metastatic cancers of the bone will be noted with hot spots and an increase of dye.

The test is ordered to help evaluate or diagnose a bone tumor or cancer, an infection of the bone, a fracture, Paget's disease (metabolic bone disorder), and unexplained causes of bone pain.

Ultrasound

Diagnostic ultrasound, also called sonography, is an imaging method that uses high-frequency sound waves to produce images of structures within the body. The procedure uses a transducer, which is placed on skin that has been treated with ultrasound gel. The transducer produces high-frequency sound waves that enter the body and are sent back to the transducer; the transducer then relays the information to a computer, which analyzes the information and creates an image. The information is helpful for diagnosing and treating a variety of diseases as well as evaluating a fetus for growth or structural problems. The test uses no radiation. The test is also frequently used to evaluate the blood flow in vessels to assess for a blood clot and to diagnose gallbladder disease. The test is typically noninvasive, but special transducers exist that can be inserted into the esophagus to get a better view of the heart, into a male's rectum to get images of the prostate, and also into a woman's vagina to evaluate her uterus and ovaries.

It is also used to see internal body structures such as tendons, muscles, joints, vessels, and internal organs, and it may be used to assist in anatomical identification for injections into these areas.

MRI

MRI is a test that uses a magnetic field and radio waves. The information is processed by a computer, which then produces very detailed images of structures inside the body. Since the test uses a magnetic field, patients with implanted pacemakers and other metal devices may not be able to have an MRI. Additionally, construction workers and welders may need to be screened before having an MRI to ensure that they do not

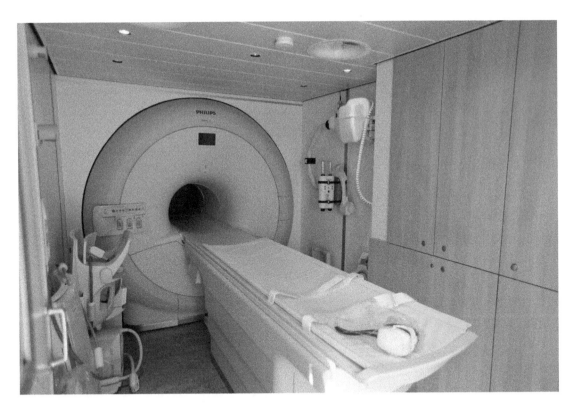

FIGURE 12.3   MRI Scanner.

have metal fragments within the eyes. MRI is safe for pregnant women, as it does not utilize radiation.

For an MRI test, the area of the body being studied is placed inside a tube that contains a strong magnet. Patients who have claustrophobia or difficulty being in tight spaces may require sedation to have the procedure. The MRI scan will obtain very detailed images of structures within the body; it is especially helpful in viewing soft tissues, including the brain and spinal column. The test can also be ordered to use dye or contrast material, which will be injected to provide better detail. The contrast material may be injected into the shoulder joint to better show a labral tear of the soft tissues of the shoulder joint or used for a spinal MRI to help differentiate scar tissue from a recurrent disc herniation.

The disadvantages of the test are the associated costs, which may require insurance companies and not treating physicians to approve the test to be completed. In addition, the patient will need to be relatively still in the tight tube for a period of about 45 minutes to an hour. The various imaging studies are summarized in Table 12.1.

TABLE 12.1   COMPARISON OF DIAGNOSTIC IMAGING TECHNIQUES

Test	Positives	Negatives	Costs	Uses
X-ray	Quick, easy, screening tool	Not great detail	$	Assess for fracture; evaluate lungs
CAT scan	Great for bony issues	Radiation	$$	Evaluation of stroke
Bone scan	Very sensitive for bony issues	Limited to bone problems	$$	Assessment of bone pain and infections
Ultrasound	No radiation	Cannot assess deep structures	$	Fetal assessment; assess for blood clots
MRI	No radiation	Cannot have if implanted metal	$$$	Soft tissue, brain, and spine imaging

---

NEED TO KNOW

CT scans expose the body to substantial large amounts of radiation. How much? If you compare the amount of radiation the body is exposed to with a standard chest X-ray with a chest CAT scan, it is approximately the equivalent of having 350 chest X-rays.[2] There are clear indications to have a CAT scan, such as the case to evaluate stroke patients for the presence of a bleed and in other serious medical problems. The test should be ordered if it will likely change the treatment approach and affect outcome.

References

1. Petrik, V., Apok, V., Britton, J. A., Bell, B. A., & Papadopoulos, M. C. (2006). Godfrey Hounsfield and the dawn of computed tomography. *Neurosurgery, 58*(4), 780–787.
2. McCollough, C. H., Bushberg, J. T., Fletcher, J. G., & Eckel, L. J. (2015). Answers to common questions about the use and safety of CT scans. *Mayo Clinic Proceedings, 90*(10), 1380–1392.

Resource

National Institute of Biomedical Imaging and Bioengineering—NIH-sponsored site that goes into nice explanations and detail of what is involved with the various imaging studies, consumer friendly site: https://www.nibib.nih.gov/science-education/science-topics/X-rays

Figure Credits

13

Dental Conditions

Objectives

▸ Understanding of the education and training of dentists and their staff
▸ Review of basic tooth anatomy
▸ Basic understanding of common dental conditions and their treatments

Dentist

The training of a dentist is not unlike that of a medical doctor. Prospective dentists will need to complete a 4-year undergraduate degree, as well as take the Dental Acceptance Test. The Associated American Dental Schools Application Service is the centralized application service for applying to U.S. dental schools. The applicants will then use the service to apply to a number of dental schools. Following the application process, they would complete an interview and await a decision from the school. If accepted, students would then need to complete 4 years of dental school. Following graduation, the degree of doctor of dental surgery (DDS) or doctor of dental medicine (DMD) would be conferred. According to the American Dental Association, there is not a difference in the training between the two degrees; some schools confer the DMD degree, while others confer the DDS degree.

Dental Hygienist

Registered dental hygienists are licensed clinicians. They may perform clinical practice procedures within their scope of practice including: performing and obtaining X-rays, removing plaque and tartar, and polishing patients' teeth. They also serve as a health educator in the office, working with the dentist to maximize patient outcomes. Dental hygienists may work in a variety of settings, including private offices, hospitals, public health clinics, and schools. Dental hygienists may be trained either in a 2-year program earning an associate's degree or a 4-year program earning a baccalaureate degree. They will need to take and successfully pass an examination for licensure to work in a dental office.

Dental Assistant

Dental assistants are another member of the dental team. These assistants will complete a 1- to 2-year training program to obtain a certification following graduation. They can further obtain a national certification following successful completion of an examination. They assist the dentist with the handling of dental instruments during procedures, preparatory tasks, taking impressions, developing radiographs, and disinfecting instruments.

Dental Specialties

Much like physicians who chose to specialize, dentists have specialty options available. Following graduation from dental school, dentists may chose additional training of 1 to 3 years to specialize. Currently, there are nine dental subspecialties that are approved by the Council on Dental Education and Licensure, American Dental Association. The specialties are dental public health, endodontics, oral and maxillofacial pathology, oral and maxillofacial radiology, oral and maxillofacial surgery, orthodontics and dentofacial orthopedics, pediatric dentistry, periodontics, and prosthodontics. Obtaining specialty certification requires completion of additional training and passing an examination.

Tooth Anatomy

The basic anatomy of a tooth is seen in Figure 13.1. The surface of the tooth is covered with the very hard and white-colored enamel. The surface gets its strength from calcium phosphate. The layer of living cells just beneath the enamel is the dentin. The inner soft structure of the tooth is the pulp. The pulp contains nerves and blood vessels.

The tissue that connects the roots of teeth to the gums and jawbone is known as cementum, and the periodontal ligament holds the teeth tightly against the jaw. The adult mouth contains 32 teeth on average. The teeth are further classified as incisors, canines, premolars, and molars. Humans get two sets of teeth; adult teeth, with the exception of the wisdom teeth, erupt and are present typically by age 13. The wisdom teeth will typically erupt around age 18. Dentists treat a number of conditions that may arise in the mouth involving the teeth and jaw.

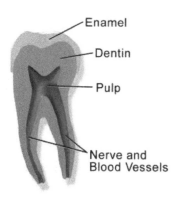

FIGURE 13.1   Tooth Anatomy.

Halitosis

Halitosis is the official name for bad breath. It has a number of causes, including the food that was eaten as well as poor oral hygiene and underlying gum disease. Bacteria are also believed to play a role in halitosis. Underlying medical conditions can also be associated with this problem and include diabetes, liver disease, and acid reflux. The problem can be prevented or treated with good oral hygiene, avoiding dehydration, and chewing sugarless gum, all of which may address the underlying cause.

Tooth Sensitivity

Tooth sensitivity is another common dental problem. It is characterized by sharp pain that is associated with exposed dentin. Pain-inducing stimuli may include those of a thermal, chemical, or tactile nature. The cause of tooth sensitivity is related to erosion or abrasion of the enamel layer. The problem is treated with desensitizing agents. These agents include fluoride rinses and toothpastes with high fluoride levels. It is also recommended to avoid acidic food, brush the teeth twice daily, and floss between the teeth and gums.

Plaque

Plaque is the term given to a sticky, colorless film of bacteria that adheres to the surface of the teeth. Bacteria that live in the mouth interact with proteins and food by-products, leading to the formation of dental plaque. It is caused by lack of proper dental care and is associated with carbohydrates (simple sugars). Prevention includes regular dental checkups, emphasizing oral hygiene, and brushing and flossing the teeth. Eating a more balanced diet and decreasing one's carbohydrate intake will also be helpful. The concern with plaque is that it will lead to damage of the tooth enamel surface, promoting tooth decay and eventually cavities. When plaque stays on the teeth and harden, this is known as tartar. The main concern with tartar is this buildup has the potential for permanent tooth decay and gum disease.

Tooth Decay

Tooth decay, also known as dental cavities or the scientific name dental caries, is caused by the bacteria buildup of plaque and tartar. The caries are most commonly found on the flat surfaces of the teeth, particularly the molars. They may be associated with pain. Prevention is consistent with good oral hygiene, including brushing and flossing and also the use of sealants and topical fluoride. If left untreated, teeth can fracture or get infected. The infection may involve the pulp or more significantly result in a painful abscess. Treatment is directed at restoration and, depending on the extent of the problem, may involve placement of a dental crown or cap over the tooth or a root canal procedure.

The root canal procedure involves removal of the damaged and infected pulp. This region is then cleaned out and prepared. The pulp is filled with gutta percha.[1] This rigid latex material is found in the sap of the Palaquium gutta tree. The material is then heated and compressed into the canal(s) of the tooth and then is sealed with adhesive cement.

Gingivitis

Gingivitis is an inflammation of the gums. It may be caused by plaque buildup as well as irritation of the gum lining. Smoking and the rubbing of dental appliances in the mouth are other causes. Drugs such as anticonvulsants (anti-seizure) medications, oral contraceptives, and steroids are also associated with gingivitis. Prevention includes good oral hygiene and avoidance of smoking. If the problem is left untreated, it will lead to the bleeding of gums with brushing, persistent halitosis, and loosening of teeth. There is also evidence that untreated gingivitis may increase the risk of a heart attack or stroke and make control of blood glucoses more difficult in diabetic patients.[2-3]

The problem may initially be treated with an antibiotic wash, dental scaling, and root planing. Dental scaling involves hand instruments to physically remove the tartar buildup on the surface of the teeth, especially at the edge of the gum line. Root planing is the use of the tool into the top portion of the gums to remove tartar. The scaling and planing procedures can also be done with ultrasonic instruments.

Oral Cancer

Oral cancers may involve the lips, tongue, and lining of the mouth and throat. Mouth cancers typically start in the squamous lining. This is the lining of the inside of the mouth. These cancers are known as squamous cell carcinomas. The causes of oral cancers are alcohol, tobacco use (both smoking and smokeless), and human papilloma virus (HPV). HPV is the most common sexually transmitted disease (STD). The incidence of oral cancers is on the rise in the United States, particularly among young white males and females since 1984—this despite general population reductions in tobacco and alcohol use.[4] The increased incidence may be secondary to the spread of HPV into the oral cavity during sex.[5] If left untreated, this cancer will spread.

Symptoms that may suggest oral cancer include a red- or white-colored patch in the mouth, a mouth sore that does not go away, or an area of pain and/or bleeding in the mouth. These concerns should promptly be brought

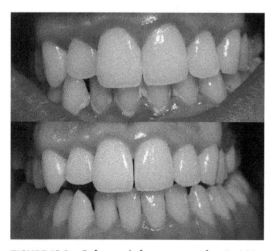

FIGURE 13.2 Before and after treatment for gingivitis.

to the attention of your dentist or physician. Treatments for oral cancers may include resection of the lesion, radiation treatments, and chemotherapy.

Teeth Grinding (Bruxism)

Bruxism is the condition in which one grinds or clenches the teeth. It can occur during the day (awake bruxism) or when one is sleeping (sleep bruxism). Sleep bruxism is considered a sleep-related movement disorder. It can result in fracturing, loosening, or loss of teeth. Stress and anxiety are related to sleep bruxism, and the presence of either type of bruxism increases the likelihood of the other type.[6-7] Treatments can involve the use of a mouth guard, avoidance of caffeine prior to bedtime, and physical therapy of the muscles of the jaw.

NEED TO KNOW

Occasionally, in the spirit of a backyard football game, a tooth may get knocked out. What to do? If the tooth is loose, it can be pushed back into place, and a dentist should be consulted. If the tooth is knocked out, it may be carefully handled, avoiding contact with the pulp end of the tooth. It can then be placed in a small, clean container. There are commercial products and solutions available to place a tooth in. Most people do not anticipate such an event; in that case the tooth can be placed in a small cup and submerged with milk or saliva from the person. The dentist should then be called, as the tooth may be able to be placed back into the socket.

References

1. Johnson, W. B. (1978). A new gutta-percha technique. *Journal of Endodontics, 4*(6), 184–188.
2. Taylor, G., & Borgnakke, W. (2008). Periodontal disease: Associations with diabetes, glycemic control and complications. *Oral Diseases, 14*, 191–203. doi:10.1111/j.1601-0825.2008.01442
3. Thorstensson, H., Kuylenstiema, J., & Hugoson, A. (1996). Medical status and complications in relation to periodontal disease experience in insulin-dependent diabetics. *Journal of Clinical Periodontology, 23*, 194–202. doi:10.1111/j.1600-051X.1996.tb02076.x
4. Tota, J. E., Anderson, W. F., et al. (2017). Rising incidence of oral tongue cancer among White men and women in the United States, 1973–2012. *Oral Oncology, 67*, 146–152.
5. Jiang, S., & Dong, Y. (2017). Human papillomavirus and oral squamous cell carcinoma: A review of HPV-positive oral squamous cell carcinoma and possible strategies for future. *Current Problems in Cancer, 41*(5), 323–327.
6. Manfredini, D., & Lobbezoo, F. (2009). Role of psychosocial factors in the etiology of bruxism. *Journal of Orofacial Pain, 23*(2), 153–166.
7. Castroflorio, T., Bargellini, A., Rossini, G., Cugliari, G., & Deregibus, A. (2017). Sleep bruxism in adolescents: A systematic literature review of related risk factors. *European Journal of Orthodontics, 39*(1), 61–68. doi:10.1093/ejo/cjw012

Resources

American Dental Association—Home of the ADA, which serves to advance dentistry care on the national and local levels, they also will approve products with the ADA seal of approval to provide consumers with reassurance and a level of quality: www.ada.org

American Dental Education Association—The National organization responsible for dental education, the site to go to find information of dental education and resources to apply to dental schools: www.adea.org

Figure Credits

14

Medical Diagnosis II

Objective

▶ Basic understanding of some common medical conditions and their appropriate management

Introduction

It has been said that the goal of the first 2 years of medical school is to learn the language of medicine and the last 2 years to learn how to treat diseases and patients. This is obviously an oversimplification, but it makes the point that medical terms and concepts can be difficult for the layperson to follow or understand. The purpose of this and subsequent chapters, which provide an overview of medical and surgical problems, is to educate the public in various common diseases and ailments. By getting a better understanding of the disease process, diagnosis and treatments should become easier to understand.

Gastroesophageal Reflux Disease

Gastroesophageal reflux disease (GERD) is the most common gastrointestinal disorder of the esophagus.[1] GERD is more prevalent in developed countries. In the United States the prevalence rate for GERD is 28.8% of the population.[2] The prevalence rate also increases with age and affects mainly adults aged from 50 to 70 years of age.

When we chew food, we propel the food bolus to the back of our mouth, and the food enters the esophagus. This is the tube that connects the mouth to the stomach. Between the esophagus and stomach is a muscle. This muscle is specifically known as a sphincter. The sphincter is actively contracting and is in the closed position. When the food bolus stretches (distends) the end of the esophagus, this signals the sphincter muscle to relax, which allows the food to enter the stomach. The stomach produces and secretes strong acids

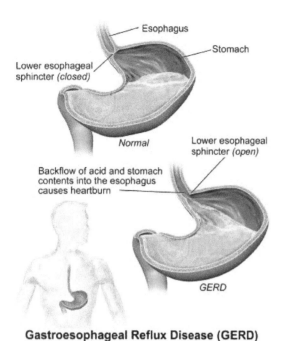

Gastroesophageal Reflux Disease (GERD)

FIGURE 14.1   Gastroesophageal Reflux Disease (GERD).

to help digest the food. The partially digested food will eventually enter the first part of the small intestine (duodenum).

The problem with GERD is that the stomach contents and juices may reflux, or enter into the esophagus. Because of the acidic nature of these fluids, they can cause an irritation to the skin of the lower region of the esophagus. This irritation can result in a number of symptoms. One may perceive a burning sensation in the chest (heartburn). This sensation may sometimes spread to the jaw. Other times a sour taste may be present in the mouth. Reflux can also cause difficulty swallowing and be associated with a dry cough. The pain sensation is very uncomfortable, and it may be difficult to pinpoint the exact location of the pain.

There are certain risk factors for the development of GERD. These include obesity, hiatal hernia in which part of the stomach migrates through the diaphragm muscle, pregnancy, smoking, and diabetes.

Certain foods have also been linked to reflux. Caffeinated beverages, chocolate, and alcohol are known to relax the esophageal sphincter. Acidic-based foods such as orange and tomato juice can also bring about symptoms. And spicy foods may also be best to avoid with ongoing problems of reflux.

Initial treatments for the problem of reflux include a glass of milk to try to neutralize the stomach acids. Avoidance of eating food late at night is also beneficial. Trying to remain upright after eating or with an incline in bed may also help. Medications are another option for individuals with GERD. The medications work by trying to neutralize the stomach acids or limit the amount of acid production. Some medications are available over the counter, while others require a prescription.

Medications such as antacids work by trying to neutralize the stomach acids including: Tums® and Rolaids®. Antacids may be purchased over the counter. There are two types of medications that work by reducing the production of stomach acids. The first group is known as H2 blockers (the is for "histamine"); these work by blocking histamine receptors in the stomach cells, thereby inhibiting gastric secretions. They work in about an hour and will last for about 8 to 12 hours. Zantac, Pepcid, Tagamet, and Axid are examples of H2 blockers. The other group of medications blocks stomach pumps that produce the acid. These are known as proton pump inhibitors. This group includes Prilosec, Protonix, and Nexium. Both groups are available over the counter and with prescriptions. The prescription dosing is at a higher strength (milligrams).

Concussion

A concussion is a mild traumatic brain injury. It is usually caused by a blow to the head in which there is a jarring or shearing force. The injury may result in the head being quickly moved in one direction and then the other. The force results in a loss of brain function. The extent of the injury and loss of function can vary greatly among individuals.

Rates of concussion are difficult to know exactly, since the diagnosis is still believed to be underreported. The rates of concussion do vary among age groups, gender, and the sport of the participant. They are common in collision sports but can occur in contact sports as well.

Recent studies have shown the overall mean rate of concussions to be 3.78 per 100,000 in youths aged 5–19 years and 0.36 per 100,000 adults.[4] Findings also noted that 75% of concussions diagnosed in this study were in males. Additional studies have evaluated the rate of concussions associated with sports at the high school and collegiate levels. Among the high school population, the incidence rate was found to be 9.2 per 10,000 for football, followed by boys' lacrosse at 6.65 per 10,000 and girls' soccer at 6.11 per 10,000.[5] Collegiate concussion studies have found that football players have an overall mean rate of concussions (4.46 per 1,000 Athletic Events (AEs), when compared to other sports women's softball (8.82/10,000 AEs), women's field hockey (7.71/10000 AEs), and men's baseball (7.20/10,000 AEs).[6-7] The relative incidences are summarized in Table 14.1.

After a concussion occurs, individuals may or may not lose consciousness. Additionally, they may have difficulty remembering where they are or have other problems with orientation. They can experience a myriad of symptoms. The most commonly reported symptoms among athletes following a concussion were headache (94.7%), dizziness (74.8%), and difficulty concentrating (61.0%).[5] Additional symptoms such as blurred vision, slowed processing, balance problems, memory issues, emotional changes, and aversion to light have been reported. It is important to remember that the symptoms can and do vary among individuals who experience a concussion. Sometimes balance may be more affected in one individual and memory and processing in another individual.

TABLE 14.1   RELATIVE CONCUSSION RATES

Population	Incidence per 10,000	Reference
General youth	0.38	Amoo-Achampong et al. (2017)
General adult	0.04	Amoo-Achampong et al. (2017)
High school football	9.2	O'Connor et al. (2017)
Collegiate football	44.6	Houck et al. (2016)
Collegiate softball	8.82	Fraser et al. (2017)
Collegiate baseball	7.20	Fraser et al. (2017)

Initial treatment following a concussion is to rest. If the concussion occurs in an athletic event, the athlete needs to be removed immediately from the competition. Sideline trainers and medical staff should be educated in the signs and symptoms of a concussion. They should take the athlete to the sideline for evaluation. The Sport Concussion Assessment Tool, 3rd edition (SCAT3™) is a standardized tool for evaluating concussed athletes older than age 13. It consists of eight sections to assess: arousal, orientation, symptoms, cognitive processing, neck movement, balance, coordination, and delayed memory. Each section is scored to assist in the diagnosis and assessment of the severity of the injury.

Following the assessment, a specific protocol for concussions may be followed. Most initial treatment involves rest. A CAT scan is not routinely recommended following a concussion unless the patient exhibits a focal neurologic deficit, such as right leg weakness or partial loss of vision. Rest is recommended in order not to overstimulate the injured brain. The concept is very similar to the treatment following a fracture. One would not be expected to try to use a broken arm just after a fracture; instead, the fracture is treated with a cast and is given 4 to 6 weeks of rest to heal. Most concussions will resolve within 1 week. Factors associated with a longer recovery period include a history of prior concussion, a lengthy period of loss of consciousness at the time of the concussion, and a history of headaches. A good indicator of recovery is improvement in symptoms. Some high school and collegiate programs will perform memory and processing testing on their athletes prior to the start of the season. The same tests will be repeated following a concussion, with allowing athletes to begin a return to play protocol when the testing is within 90% of their initial baseline testing. The return to play protocol is a gradual 5- to 7-day process, with increasing activities and exercise challenges. If an athlete remains symptom free during the challenges, he or she may advance to the next step in the protocol. If the athlete develops symptoms, he or she should reduce the activity to the next lower level in the protocol.

Medicine does not have all of the answers today when it comes to concussions. We certainly know more about the treatment and consequences of concussions then was known 10 years ago. Given that understanding, it may be prudent to error on the side of caution and conservative treatment when treating a concussion.

Multiple Sclerosis

Multiple sclerosis (MS) is a disease of the central nervous system associated with neurological findings and a clinical course that shows variation. MS involves an immune-mediated process in which an abnormal response of the body's immune system is directed at the central nervous system. The disease involves a disruption of the signals or flow of the information in the central nervous system. The central nervous system is composed of the brain, spinal cord, and cranial nerves. The exact antigen the immune cells are sensitized to remains unknown, possibly a virus. Nonetheless, the body will be producing antibodies against structures in its own central nervous system; for this reason the disease is referred to as immune mediated. Currently, the exact cause of the disease is unknown but thought to be triggered in a genetically susceptible individual by a combination of one or more environmental factors.

According to the National Multiple Sclerosis Society, in the United States the number of people with MS is estimated to be about 400,000, with approximately 10,000 new cases diagnosed every year (that's 200 new cases per week). MS is much more common in females than males. Most cases of MS are diagnosed in people aged 20 to 50. The diagnosis is made on clinical grounds, meaning the physician, usually a neurologist, will take into account the history of symptoms and physical examination findings. Certain tests can be ordered to confirm the diagnosis. An MRI of the brain or spinal cord can show demyelinating lesions. A nerve conduction/electromyography study will be normal but may be helpful in ruling out peripheral nerve problems that could be causing extremity (limb) numbness. Lumbar puncture with analysis of the cerebral spinal fluid and electrophysiological tests of vision may also assist in the diagnosis. The average age when MS symptoms first appear is between 30 and 35. The disease is also more common among people in Europe, the United States, and Canada. The incidence of disease increases as one moves farther from the equator.

Nerves within our central nervous system are covered with a coating called myelin. Myelin insulates the nerves and enables the transmission of impulses to travel at a faster speed. In MS the immune system attacks the myelin within the central nervous system. The damaged myelin forms scar tissue (sclerosis), which gives the disease its name. The attacks can be in multiple areas of the central nervous system; hence, the use of in naming the disease.

When any part of the myelin sheath or nerve fiber is damaged or destroyed, nerve impulses traveling to and from the brain and spinal cord are distorted or interrupted, producing a wide variety of symptoms. The symptoms depend on the exact location of the disrupted signals. Common symptoms seen with MS include optic neuritis (visual problems with vision blurring), extremity (limb) numbness, fatigue, emotional lability, weakness, and pain.

The course of the disease may be progressive or may wax and wane. The symptoms and functional disabilities may show fluctuations more on a long-term basis rather than on a daily or hourly basis. Treatments for MS are available and include medications and therapies. Unfortunately, no medications or treatments exist that will cure MS, but they will help treat the symptoms associated with MS. The medications in general are directed at modulating the immune response of the body. Recently, medications have shown some promise in decreasing the frequency of the relapse of symptoms, include Avonex, Betaseron, and Copaxone.

The medications Avonex and Betaseron are genetically produced proteins which mimics the action of interferon beta. Interferon beta, which is produced by the body, has antiviral actions and helps regulate the immune response. The exact mechanism of this protein is unknown. The medication is taken once a week via injection into a muscle. Copaxone is a synthetic protein that works by simulating myelin. Myelin is the protein that is damaged by the T cells of the immune system. The mechanism by which this works is not completely understood. Copaxone can be injected either daily or three times a week.

Therapies may be ordered to address weakness and neurologic problems. Physical therapy can be ordered by a physician to improve weakness and maximize function in individuals with MS. Therapists may also be able to train patients to use assistive devices (e.g., a walker or cane) to maintain mobility. In addition, they can outline a home exercise program to maintain strength and minimize stiffness.

NEED TO KNOW

Red Flag

A red flag warning is issued by the National Weather Service when conditions are met that could lead to a wildfire. The red flag is placed out of concern. In medicine, a symptom described by a patient can be indicative of an underlying serious medical problem. Such concerns are known as medical red flags. Physicians will ask patients about symptoms that could indicate a significant underlying problem. Some symptoms in patients that are red flags include unexplained weight loss, night sweats, persistent fevers, and back pain at night. Any of these symptoms will warrant additional questioning and potentially additional testing.

References

1. Kethman, W., & Hawn, M. (2017). New approaches to gastroesophageal reflux disease. *Journal of Gastrointestinal Surgery*. doi:10.1007/s11605-017-3439-5

2. Ronkainen, J., & Agréus, L. (2013). Epidemiology of reflux symptoms and GORD. *Best Practice & Research Clinical Gastroenterology, 27*(3), 325–337. doi:10.1016/j.bpg.2013.06.008

3. Savarino, E., Marabotto, E., et al. (2017). Epidemiology and natural history of gastro-esophageal reflux disease. *Minerva Gastroenterologica e Dietololgica*. doi:10.23736/S1121-421X.17.02383-2

4. Amoo-Achampong, K., Rosas, S., et al. (2017). Trends in sports-related concussion diagnoses in the USA: A population-based analysis using a private-payor database. *Physician and Sportsmedicine*, 1–6. doi:10.1080/00913847.2017.1327304

5. O'Connor, K. L., Baker, M. M., Dalton, S. L., Dompier, T. P., Broglio, S. P., & Kerr Z. Y. (2017). Epidemiology of sport-related concussions in high school athletes: National Athletic Treatment, Injury and Outcomes Network (NATION), 2011–2012 Through 2013–2014. *Journal of Athletic Training, 52*(3), 175–185. doi:10.4085/1062-6050-52.1.15

6. Houck, Z., Asken, B., Bauer, R., Pothast, J., Michaudet, C., & Clugston, J. (2016). Epidemiology of sport-related concussion in an NCAA Division I football bowl subdivision sample. *American Journal of Sports Medicine, 44*(9), 2269–2275. doi:10.1177/0363546516645070

7. Fraser, M. A., Grooms, D. R., Guskiewicz, K. M, & Kerr, Z. Y. (2017). Ball-contact injuries in 11 National Collegiate Athletic Association sports: The Injury Surveillance Program, 2009–2010 Through 2014–2015. *Journal of Athletic Training.* doi:10.4085/1062-6050-52.3.10

Figure Credit

15

Surgical Diagnosis II

Objective

▸ Basic understanding of some common surgical conditions and their appropriate management

Introduction

For a better understanding of this chapter, it is probably best to start with a few medical terms and their definitions. When **is** attached to the end of a word, it denotes inflammation. Examples are neuritis (nerve inflammation), gastritis (stomach irritation/inflammation), and arthritis (joint inflammation). When taking a history of a patient, the patient may describe sensations or pains he or she is having; these descriptions are known as symptoms. A sign is a finding that is present on physical examination. A mnemonic device for remembering this is: "**I**" the physician describe the s**I**gn and "**Y**ou" the patient describe the s**Y**mptom.

Appendicitis

Appendicitis is a surgical emergency. In the United States 1 in 15 people will get appendicitis. Although it can strike at any age, appendicitis is rare under age 2 and most common between ages 10 and 30. A life table model suggests that the lifetime risk of appendicitis is 8.6% for males and 6.7% for females.[1] Chances are you likely know someone who has experienced appendicitis.

Appendicitis occurs when the appendix becomes blocked, often by stool, a foreign body, or a tumor. Blockage may also occur from infection, since the appendix swells in response to any infection in the body. The urgency related to the problem can occur if the swelled appendix ruptures. The ruptured contents of the appendix can expose the peritoneum (abdominal cavity) to bacteria and the potential for a life-threatening emergency.

The patient will describe certain symptoms that are suggestive of appendicitis. The earliest symptom may begin as periumbilical (around the belly button) or epigastric pain. The pain over time will localize to the right lower quadrant of the abdomen. Pain in the right lower quadrant of the abdomen is classic for appendicitis. Nausea is also a common symptom, occurring in 61%–92% of patients, and anorexia (loss of appetite for food) in about 75% of patients.[1] Vomiting nearly always follows the onset of pain. If the vomiting precedes pain, it suggests intestinal obstruction.

Diarrhea or constipation are less common symptoms that can be described. Another classic finding is fever, or an elevated temperature of typically greater than 100°F (normal body temperature is 98.6°F).

Physical examination signs that the patient will exhibit include abdominal pain with guarding and rebound tenderness. The abdominal pain may be diffuse (throughout) or localized to the right lower quadrant of the abdomen. The patient may also exhibit guarding; this describes a reluctance to move that region of the abdomen. Another sign that is suggestive of appendicitis is rebound tenderness. This sign is elicited when the lower portion of the abdomen is pushed and then released. The patient will describe an increase in pain not during the compressive push, but the release or rebound of the abdominal wall.

To assist in the diagnosis, additional studies can confirm the suspicions. Laboratory blood studies include obtaining a CBC and a c-reactive protein (for a lab test that measures inflammation or infection in the body). Both of the labs will demonstrate marked elevations. Imaging studies may also help confirm the diagnosis. These studies include an abdominal ultrasound, which may show swelling and inflammation of the appendix. An abdominal CT scan can also confirm an enlarged or ruptured appendix. MRI would be the imaging study of choice in pregnant women, as it does not utilize radiation. In pediatric patients, American College of Emergency Physicians (ACEP) clinical policy recommends ultrasonography for confirmation, but not exclusion, of acute appendicitis. To definitively exclude acute appendicitis, the ACEP recommends a CT scan.

There are a few diagnoses in medicine that do not require making a choice among treatments. Appendicitis is one of them; it requires surgery. The surgery can either be done by an open approach or via a laparoscopic approach. The open approach may be necessary in the case of a ruptured appendix to allow for better viewing and access to the peritoneal cavity, which will require irrigation and removal of infected tissue and bowel contents.

Postoperatively, the patient will be maintained on antibiotics until the patient is afebrile (without fever) and his or her WBC count normalizes. Pregnant patients will receive category A or B antibiotics.

Rotator Cuff Tendinitis

Rotator cuff tendinitis refers to inflammation or microtears to the tendons of the rotator cuff muscles of the shoulder. Tendons, which are found throughout the human body, are a strong band of connective tissue that connects a muscle to a bone. The rotator cuff describes a set of four muscles in the shoulder region. The muscles work to lift the arm and hand away from the body as well as rotate the shoulder. The shoulder may be rotated internally or externally. The supraspinatus, infraspinatus, teres minor, and subscapularis are the four muscles that make up the rotator cuff. [Fig. 15.1]

When the muscles are weak and overworked, there is a potential for the tendon to be damaged. The damage may result in inflammation of the tendon leading to pain with movement or progress to a small tear leading to tendinosis. Either will make movement or activation of the rotator cuff muscles painful, weak, or limited in terms of movement. The medical term for movement of a particular muscle or joint is range of motion (ROM). The patient may also report difficulty sleeping on that side of the body secondary to pain in the shoulder. The pain caused by a rotator cuff tends to occur at the edge of the shoulder and may radiate toward the elbow. Classically, rotator cuff pain does not radiate below the elbow. Pain in the shoulder that radiates into the wrist or hand is more suggestive of nerve pain, with compression points being in the shoulder or in the neck.

Risk factors for rotator cuff tendinitis are male gender, increased age, and occupations that require heavy lifting. Initial treatments for rotator cuff tendinitis are conservative and involve physical therapy, medications, and injections. Surgery is reserved for refractory cases.

The physician may order physical therapy in an effort to improve the pain and reduced ROM associated with rotator cuff tendinitis. The physical therapy prescription should focus on restoring the impaired ROM. This can be done with an emphasis on stretching of the posterior capsule of the shoulder. Strengthening of the rotator cuff muscles may also be addressed. Typically, to strengthen muscles weights are lifted to provide increasing resistance. However, the rotator cuff muscles are very thin, and heavy weights would likely tear them. The therapist will employ the use of TheraBands®. These are strips of latex

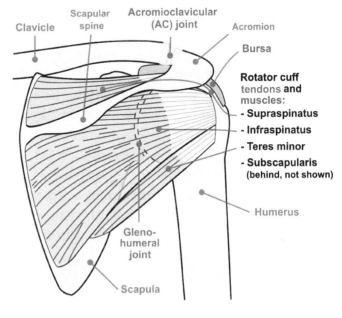

FIGURE 15.1 Rotator Cuff Muscles.

bands that come in a variety of strengths or elasticity and in different colors. The therapist will then instruct the patient on a strengthening program using the bands.

Medications to reduce inflammation can also be used; this group of medications includes anti-inflammatories. This class of medications is available OTC or can be obtained with a physician's prescription for higher doses. If medications and therapies are not effective, injections of medications into the shoulder region may be helpful. Steroids, which are very strong anti-inflammatory medications, are used and are fairly effective. It is recommended that the number of steroid injections be limited to no more than three times a year in the same joint.

Occasionally, the patient fails conservative treatments as outlined previously, and surgery is the only option left. The surgery is more commonly done via an arthroscopic approach and may entail repairing the torn muscles/tendons, removing torn tissues and arthritic bony buildup, to provide more room relieving a potential impingement of the tissues. Following surgery, the patient will follow a postoperative protocol directed by the orthopedic surgeon and carried out by a physical therapist.

Carpal Tunnel Syndrome

Carpal tunnel syndrome involves compression of the median nerve at the region of the wrist, more specifically in the carpal tunnel. The median nerve is one of the two main nerves of the hand, the ulnar nerve being the other one. They are each responsible for providing sensation to the surface of the hand, and each account for about half of the motor strength of the hand muscles.

Carpal tunnel syndrome is the most common entrapment neuropathy, affecting approximately 3% to 6% of adults in the general population; [2] other studies estimate the prevalence to be 14.4%.[3]

The carpal tunnel is the anatomical space formed by the carpal bones of the hand. The tunnel contains the flexor tendons of the hand as well as the median nerve. The roof of the tunnel is formed by the transverse carpal ligament (flexor retinaculum). The median nerve gets compressed in the tunnel. The median nerve supplies sensory nerves to most fingers of the hand. These digits include the thumb, index, middle, and half of the ring finger. The ulnar nerve, which is not in the carpal tunnel, supplies sensation to the remaining half of the ring finger and the entire little finger.

Individuals who have carpal tunnel syndrome will describe a number of symptoms. The most common is a complaint of numbness of the hand; most patients describe the entire hand, though typically the little finger will not truly be numb. In addition, patients may describe weakness with grip strength of the hand and occasional dropping of objects. They may also be awakened in the night with numbness, often shaking the hand out. Some patients will describe the sensation more in terms of a feeling of impaired blood flow to the hand. The blood flow to the hand is not the problem; as this sensation is produced secondary to the compression of the median nerve. Patients may also describe the fingers of the hand feeling swollen.

The cause of the problem is compression of the median nerve. The compression may be the result of trauma or arthritis to the carpal tunnel region. Additional risk factors associated with an increased incidence of carpal tunnel syndrome include diabetes, pregnancy, and hypothyroidism.

The history and physical examination should support the diagnosis. The physical examination of the patient may reveal numbness of the thumb, index, middle, and ring fingers of the hand. In addition, there may be weakness of certain muscles of the fingers and thumb.

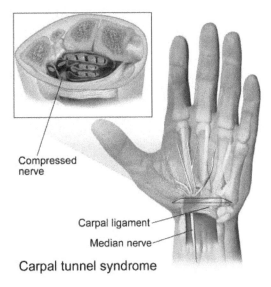

Carpal tunnel syndrome

FIGURE 15.2 Carpal Tunnel Syndrome.

Tapping on the nerve with a reflex hammer at the carpal tunnel may illicit symptoms of tingling in the hand. Reproduction of nerve symptoms with testing is known as a "Tinel's test." The diagnosis can then be confirmed by an electrodiagnostic study. The electrodiagnostic test will stimulate nerves in the hand, wrist, and carpal tunnel; the speed of the nerves will be delayed and possibly the size of the nerve responses will be reduced. This test may also be able to determine the severity of the carpal tunnel syndrome, usually on the basis of mild, moderate, and severe. The patients in the moderate category tend to have the best outcomes with surgical release. Those in the mild group have limited compression present to benefit from a release, and those in the severe group may have damage that will not improve following a surgical release.

The initial treatment for the mild and the moderate group is to use a neutral resting wrist splint at night. This helps maintain the wrist in a neutral position throughout the night. The neutral position of the wrist places the least amount of pressure on the median nerve in the carpal tunnel; flexion of the wrist will promote a compression force on the nerve and extension will promote a stretching force at the wrist.

Surgical release of the transverse carpal ligament may be necessary to resolve the problem. The surgery is better described as a procedure. It is done on an outpatient basis. The procedure does not require general anesthesia and can be done under local anesthesia. It typically takes 15 minutes to perform. The recovery following the procedure is directed by the surgeon and will depend on the surgeon's protocols and the finding at the time of the release. The surgical success rate approaches 97%. In patients with severe symptoms, including weakness, it is best not to delay having the release done, since persistent nerve compression can lead to irreversible symptoms.

References

1. Addiss, D. G., Shaffer, N., Fowler, B. S., & Tauxe, R. V. (1990). The epidemiology of appendicitis and appendectomy in the United States. *American Journal of Epidemiology, 132*(5), 910–925.
2. LeBlanc, K. E., & Cestia, W. (2011). Carpal tunnel syndrome. *American Family Physician, 83*(8), 952–958.
3. Atroshi, I., Gummesson, C., et al. (1999). Prevalence of carpal tunnel syndrome in a general population. *Journal of the American Medical Association, 282*(2), 153–158. doi:10.1001/jama.282.2.153

Figure Credits

16

Nutrition Principles

Objectives

- ▸ Basic understanding of caloric intake and weight gain
- ▸ Review of caloric expenditures
- ▸ Review of caloric intake
- ▸ Brief review of healthy eating

Nutrition

Nutrition is defined by Oxford Dictionaries as the process of providing or obtaining the food necessary for health and growth. The food we ingest provides the body with energy to grow and maintain itself. Food energy is denoted in terms of calories, a measurement of energy. We can think of calories as both consumed and expended or burned. One's diet is made up of the calories consumed, and the calories burned relates to one's activity.

Calories are denoted in terms of kilocalories (kcal), and 1 kilocalorie is equal to 1,000 calories. The food we ingest contains calories, which are based on the structure and components of the food. This is referred to as input. The amount of energy we expend can be thought of as output. If our input is greater than our output, we gain weight, and if our output is greater than our input, we lose weight. When our intake or input exceeds our output, our body converts the calories into fat.

One pound of fat is equivalent to 3,500 calories. So if an individual's intake for the week is 3,500 calories higher than his/her output, the person will gain 1 pound of weight. The pound of weight in nongrowing adults is added to the body as fat. Fat is used by our body to store excess energy, which can be burned at a later time if needed. This becomes a problem when excess fat is not burned and additional fat continues to get added. In the United States obesity rates are on the rise. Obesity in medical terms is defined as a body mass index greater than 30. The body mass index can be calculated based on a person's height and weight. Body mass index ranges are presented in Table 16.1.

TABLE 16.1   HARRIS BENEDICT EQUATION TO DETERMINE BMR[2]

Male BMR = 88.362 + (13.397 × weight (kg)) + (4.799 × height (cm)) + (5.677 × age (yrs))

Female BMR = 447.593 + (9.247 × weight (kg)) + (3.098 × height (cm)) + (4.33 × age (yrs))

In order to lose 1 pound of weight (fat) in a week, your weekly intake needs to decrease by 3,500 calories. That breaks down to a difference of 500 calories a day. You must take in 500 calories less a day or expend 500 calories more in a day, or some combination of the two.

Output

There are three ways the body will expend energy: basal metabolic rate, thermic effect of food, and physical activity or exercise.

Basal Metabolic Rate

The basal metabolic rate (BMR) is the amount of energy needed to maintain a resting state and carry out the basic metabolic functions of the body. This energy expenditure is when the body is at rest. Energy is required to maintain your body at 98.6°F despite fluctuations in the ambient temperature. If you are in a hot environment, the body will need to sweat in an attempt to cool the body, which requires energy. If you are in a cold environment, the body may respond by shivering, which also involves energy. Your body needs energy to enable your lungs to breathe and your heart to beat every minute of your life.

The BMR accounts for approximately 60% of the daily energy expenditures for the day. The BMR can be calculated in the laboratory environment or estimated through mathematical formulas. Direct calorimetry is a laboratory technique in which the subject is confined to a chamber. The change in temperature after the subject enters the chamber is recorded; this change in temperature is due to the subject's energy being burned, which is measured as a change in temperature of the chamber. This technique is very accurate but requires willing subjects and appropriate equipment. Indirect calorimetry is another technique to estimate energy expenditure. It measures concentrations of expired air over a long time period. It specifically looks at carbon dioxide production and oxygen consumption during rest. This technique requires less expense and is easier than direct calorimetry, but it is less accurate.[1]

Another method to determine BMR is with the use of an equation. In 1919 scientists J. Arthur Harris and Francis G. Benedict published a formula to approximate values for BMR.[2] The formula was derived using body surface area (computed from height and weight), age, and sex, along with the oxygen and carbon dioxide measures taken from calorimetry. The formula can be reviewed in Table 16.1. Recent studies still support the accuracy of this equation nearly 100 years later.[3]

Some of the issues with weight gain are related to age. We know that as we age, our weight can easily climb. One aspect of this gain is related to the BMR. Our BMR decreases as we age. The Harris–Benedict equation subtracts age when calculating BMR. Additional studies support this change with age. One study found our total energy expenditure fell by approximately 150 kcal per decade and concluded this progressive decline in BMR and total energy expenditure has implications for defining dietary energy requirements at different stages of adult life.[4] In short, as we age one cannot eat like they did when they were younger.

Thermic Effect of Food

The thermic effect of food (TEF) is another way the body expends energy. The TEF is defined as the increase in metabolic rate after ingestion of a meal.[5] This is the energy used to digest, absorb, and metabolize food. The energy is higher for digestion of complex carbohydrates and protein than it is for fat. The TEF accounts for about 8% of the total energy expenditure. There is more energy expended when one drinks a cup of ice water compared to an equivalent amount of room temperature water, but the energy expenditure is an insignificant difference. It does not warrant drinking ice water to burn more calories and lose weight.

Exercise

The remaining way our bodies burn calories is through exercise. The exercise aspect accounts for the remaining 32% of the total energy expenditure. The amount of energy used or burned depends of the specific activity or exercise. The different types of exercises and their effects will be detailed further in the Chapter 18.

Input

The other half of the weight gain/loss balance is intake or input. This refers to the food and liquids that we consume. Each of the basic nutrients contain different calorie amounts. Carbohydrates and proteins each contain 4 calories per gram, fats 9 calories per gram, and alcohol 7 calories per gram. Alcohol is sometimes referred to as "empty calories" as it contains no nutritional value. The various nutrients are listed in Table 16.2.

TABLE 16.2   NUTRIENT COMPARISONS

Nutrient	Calories per gram
Carbohydrates	4
Protein	4
Alcohol	7
Fat	9

Carbohydrates

Carbohydrates are nutrients that provide the body with energy. They can be further divided into simple carbohydrates and complex carbohydrates. *Simple carbohydrates* are sugars. Naturally occurring sugars include glucose and fructose. The simple carbohydrates are found naturally in fruits and milk. They may also be processed into candy, syrups, and soft drinks. They are associated with a sweet taste. Refined sugars may also be thought of as "empty calories" since they contain no vitamins or minerals. Simple carbohydrates and their high glycemic index (GI) will raise blood sugar levels quicker and higher than any other type of food.

Complex carbohydrates are also known as starches. Like simple carbohydrates, complex carbohydrates are also made up of sugar molecules, although the molecules are joined in long chains. In contrast to simple carbohydrates, complex carbohydrates provide important minerals and vitamins to the diet. Complex carbohydrates, being composed of sugars, will be broken down by the body for use as energy or converted to glycogen for storage in the liver. This conversion takes a longer time and has a higher GI than simple carbohydrates.

The GI is based on the food's effect on blood glucose compared with a standard reference food. A food with a high GI raises blood glucose more than a food with a medium or low GI. According to the American Diabetes Association, meal planning with the GI involves choosing foods that have a low or medium GI. If eating a food with a high GI, you can combine it with low-GI foods to help balance the meal. Meats and fats don't have a GI because they do not contain carbohydrates.

Fiber may be found within certain complex carbohydrates. Fiber may be further broken down into soluble and insoluble types. *Soluble fiber* works to improve blood sugar levels and also helps lower cholesterol levels. It is found in beans, lentils, nuts, and oat bran. As soluble fiber passes through the digestive system, if attracts water, which helps slow digestion and soften the stool. This aids in treating constipation-related issues. *Insoluble fiber*, which is found in whole grains, vegetables, and wheat bran, also aids in digestion. Soluble and insoluble fiber cannot be digested by humans.

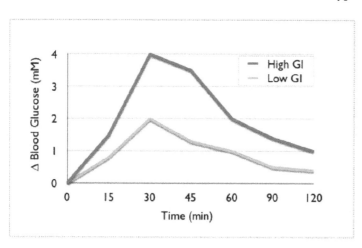

FIGURE 16.1   Impact on Blood Glucose following ingestion of a high and low glycemic foods.

Protein

Protein is found in both animal and plant sources. It is used for energy and also to help build and support the cells of the body. Protein is made up of thousands of amino acids that are chained together. The amino acids are building blocks for our muscles, skin, bones, and internal organs. Protein is also used by our body to support our immune system. It is also needed for the production of enzymes and hormones by the body. Protein is a necessary part of our diet. Foods that are sources of protein include meat, fish, chicken, eggs, milk, beans, and soy.

Fats are an essential part of our diet. Our bodies require fats to construct cell membranes, insulate nerves, produce hormones, and absorb vitamins. Fats are more difficult to digest than carbohydrates. There are two main types of fats: saturated and unsaturated. The unsaturated fats can further be subdivided into monounsaturated and polyunsaturated.

Saturated fats are found mainly in animal sources, but not exclusively. Sources may include cheese, whole milk, bacon, beef, and pork. Saturated fats tend to be solid at room temperature. They are so named because their structure does not contain any double bonds between the carbons and they are saturated with hydrogen molecules. Historically, these fats have been considered bad fats and were thought to contribute to cardiovascular disease and specifically strokes and heart attacks. However, a meta-analysis following 347,000 subjects over 5 to 23 years found no such evidence that dietary saturated fat is associated with an increased risk of coronary heart disease or cardiovascular disease.[6]

Additional studies have looked to see if any health benefits occur with a reduction of saturated fats in the diet. They were able to conclude that replacing 5% of saturated fats in one's diet with polyunsaturated fat lowers the risk of coronary artery disease by about 10%.[7] It is for this reason the American Heart Association recommends that the intake of saturated fats be limited to no more than 7% of total intake.[8]

Monounsaturated Fats

Monounsaturated fats are found in plant sources. They are liquid at room temperature but will harden if chilled. Avocados, almonds, and pumpkin seeds all contain monounsaturated fats. These fats, along with polyunsaturated fats, are considered good fats. Research has shown that partial substitution of carbohydrate with either protein or monounsaturated fat can further lower blood pressure, improve lipid levels, and reduce estimated cardiovascular risk.[9] The American Heart Association suggests that 8% to 10% of daily calories should come from polyunsaturated fats.

Polyunsaturated Fats

Polyunsaturated fats are also considered good fats. They are found in both animal and plant sources. Salmon, walnuts, and sunflower oil are all sources of polyunsaturated fats. Polyunsaturated fats are also sources of omega-3 and omega-6 fatty acids. These are both essential fatty acids that the body needs but cannot produce them its own. Omega-3 fatty acids are found specifically in fish, and omega-6 fatty acids in plant sources. Research has suggested the benefits of increasing the intake of both essential fatty acids, particularly omega-3, due to their anti-inflammatory effects.[10]

NEED TO KNOW

High fructose corn syrup has been a proposed health concern. Companies have made a point to list on their products various slogans such as "Contains NO high fructose corn syrup" or "Made with Natural Sugar." There is no significant difference between high fructose corn syrup and table sugar (sucrose). Sucrose is made up of 50% glucose and 50% fructose. High fructose corn syrup is also made up of a glucose–fructose mixture, either in a 58:42 or a 45:55 ratio. What matters more is the total amount of the sugar in the food product.

References

1. Webb, P., Annis, J. F., & Troutman, S. J., Jr. (1980). Energy balance in man measured by direct and indirect calorimetry. *American Journal of Clinical Nutrition, 33*(6), 1287–1298.
2. Harris, J. A., & Benedict, F. G. (1919). *A biometric study of basal metabolism in man.* Washington, DC: Carnegie Institution.
3. Flack, K. D., Siders, W. A., Johnson, L., & Roemmich, J. N. (2016). Cross-validation of resting metabolic rate prediction equations. *Journal of the Academy of Nutrition and Dietetics, 116*(9), 1413–1422. doi:10.1016/j.jand.2016.03.018
4. Roberts, S. B., & Dallal, G. E. (2005). Energy requirements and aging. *Public Health Nutrition, 8*(7A), 1028–1036.
5. Reed, G. W., & Hill, J. O. (1996). Measuring the thermic effect of food. *American Journal of Clinical Nutrition, 63*(2), 164–169.
6. Siri-Tarino, P. W., Sun, Q., Hu, F. B., Krauss, R. M. et al. (2010). Meta-analysis of prospective cohort studies evaluating the association of saturated fat with cardiovascular disease. *American Journal of Clinical Nutrition, 91*(3), 535–546.
7. Micha, R., & Mozaffarian, D. (2010). Saturated fat and cardiometabolic risk factors, coronary heart disease, stroke, and diabetes: A fresh look at the evidence. *Lipids, 45*(10), 893–905.
8. Lichtenstein, A. H., Appel, L. J., Brands, M., Carnethon, M., et al. (2006). Diet and lifestyle recommendations revision 2006: A scientific statement from the American Heart Association Nutrition Committee. *Circulation, 114*(1), 82–96.
9. Appel, L. J., Sacks, F. M., Carey, V. J., Obarzanek, E. et al. (2005). Effects of protein, monounsaturated fat, and carbohydrate intake on blood pressure and serum lipids: Results of the OmniHeart randomized trial. *Journal of the American Medical Association, 294*(19), 2455–2464.
10. Harris, W. (2010). Omega-6 and omega-3 fatty acids: Partners in prevention. *Current Opinion in Clinical Nutrition and Metabolic Care, 13*(2), 125–129. doi:10.1097/MCO.0b013e3283357242

Resources

Nutrition.gov—is a USDA-sponsored website that offers credible information for consumers to make informed and healthful eating choices: www.nutrition.gov

American Diabetes Association—Home page of the association dedicated to informing and improving individuals and family members with diabetes: http://www.diabetes.org/

Figure Credit

Fig. 16.1: Source: https://commons.wikimedia.org/wiki/File:Glycemic.png.

17

Nutrition Choices

Objective

▸ Understanding of the options regarding making nutrition choices

Nutrition

Nutrition is the food we ingest that provides our body with the necessary energy to grow and maintain itself. Food energy is denoted in terms of calories, a measurement of energy. One pound of fat is equivalent to 3,500 calories. An individual will gain 1 pound of weight when his or her caloric intake exceeds expenditure by 3,500 calories. There are three ways the body expends energy: basal metabolic rate, thermic effect of food and through physical activity or exercise.

There is very little that can be done to change one's basal metabolic rate. The thermic effect of food is also fixed. Exercise is an expenditure variable that an individual can control. The biggest control one has over weight is the intake of food.

Concern

The rates of obesity in the United States continue to present a major medical problem for the country on a national scale. On an individual level, obesity and excessive weight are associated with a number of medical problems. Increased rates of heart disease, diabetes, high blood pressure, cancer, and arthritis are associated with obesity. A number of factors have played a role in the obesity problem. The solution to this problem needs to address multiple issues and areas of concern. Educating the public, should create a better awareness and allow for healthier choices to be made.

Education

It is important to understand the basics of calories and the calories that are associated with the foods we eat. Nobody can memorize all of the calories associated with the foods we eat. There are applications for smart phones to help with calorie counts. There has also been progress in this area in regard to chain restaurants (20 or more restaurants). According to the FDA, Americans eat and drink about 33% of their calories away from home. A statute was passed with the FDA's final rule that "nutrition labeling in chain restaurants and similar retail food establishments will provide consumers with clear and consistent nutrition information in a direct and accessible manner for the foods they eat and buy for their families."[1] This will provide consumers with information to make more informed choices about the foods they eat. The information posted will include calorie information as it relates to suggested daily caloric intake. More detailed information, including the breakdown of fats, carbohydrates, fiber, sugar, and protein, will be made available in writing on request. The original compliance date was May 2017, but this deadline was extended to May 2018.

Awareness

The caloric information should certainly help with education and awareness for the public. Knowing the information is helpful, but having a strong awareness of the information should help further. One may hear the common phrase "I know it's bad for me but . . ." What exactly does mean? Are consumers aware of what exactly bad is? And how long can we make those choices without consequences?

The focus will now be on examining what we do know about our choices and the possible consequences, in order to increase awareness. Diabetes remains a considerable health concern. The development of late-onset or type 2 diabetes is known to be related to obesity. Research has also found additional risk factors. Can drinking soda increase one's risk of developing diabetes? One study looking into this question was conducted by a group of Harvard researchers over a 9-year period and involved over 50,000 female subjects. They found women who consumed one or more sugar-sweetened soft drinks per day had a relative risk of type 2 diabetes 1.83 times greater than those who consumed less than one of these beverages per month. Similarly, consumption of fruit punch was associated with an increased diabetes risk 2.00 times greater than those who did not consume fruit punch.[2] This study was published in 2004, yet this is likely the first time most readers are becoming aware of it.

Follow-up studies have shown similar findings. A study in African American females to evaluate the risks of both soft drinks and fruit juice (which is thought to be a healthier alternative to soda) found consumption of two or more soft drinks increased the risk

	20 Years Ago		Today	
	Portion	Calories	Portion	Calories
Bagel	3″ diameter	140	6″ diameter	350
Cheeseburger	1	333	1	590
Spaghetti w/meatballs	1 cup sauce 3 small meatballs	500	cups sauce large meatballs	1,020
Soda	6.5 ounces	82	20 ounces	250
Blueberry muffin	1.5 ounces	210	5 ounces	500

of developing diabetes by 28%, and fruit juice consumption increased the risk by 30%.[3] This study was published in 2008. A more recent study from 2016, noted that adults who consume at least two (200 ml) servings of soda daily are 2.4 times more likely to develop type 2 diabetes.[4] Having the caloric information may help to some degree, but having an awareness is more likely to influence better choices.

Count

The recommended calorie needs are different from person to person. The calorie recommendations tend to be higher for males than females at the same ages. Also, calorie intake reaches its peak at ages 17 to 20 for males and ages 19 to 25 for nonpregnant females. The recommendations also depend on the daily activity levels, ranging from sedentary, moderately active, to active. The U.S. Department of Agriculture (USDA) recommendations can be reviewed in Table 17.1. This table compares the portions and calories from 20 years ago to present day.

Calorie counting can be done to know the exact daily intake of calories. Another factor to keep in mind is the caloric density of the food ingested. Certain foods are very dense with calories. These foods will contain a large amount of calories in a small amount of food. Foods that are low in calorie density will tend to be larger in size. This can help with satiety and gastric distension, giving one a feeling of being full after eating. For example, cheese has a high caloric density, while an apple has a low caloric density. One can eat a bite-sized piece of cheese or opt for two apples. Their calories are equal, but the satiety with eating one bite-sized piece of cheese is much different than two apples. Some of the recommended daily dietary recommendations account for calorie density.

Choices

Having the necessary information and awareness may not guarantee that healthier choices are made. Unfortunately, it is easier and cheaper to eat unhealthy foods than it is to eat healthy foods. Fruits and vegetables may typically involve some effort to prepare or cook, versus getting a box of processed food that can be heated in a microwave in minutes. When traveling, the options on the road or at the airport may also present a problem, as choices may be limited. Planning ahead, packing a healthy snack, and having small meals may help.

Oversize

When purchasing an item, most people are inclined to get a value or get their money's worth. When this concept is applied to food, the end result may not always be in their best interests from a health perspective. For example, certain fast-food chains and convenience stores may charge the same the price for a soft drink regardless of whether it is small, medium, large or extra-large. The price may be the same, but the calories and amount of sugar contained in the different sizes are not.

Portions have also increased over the years; what we think of as a portion now has changed dramatically. According to the National Institutes of Health:

> Some examples include a bagel 20 years ago being 3 inches in diameter and containing 140 calories. Today's bagel averages 6 inches in diameter and contains 350 calories. The average soda was 6.5 ounces and contained 82 calories; today's soda averages 20 ounces and 250 calories.

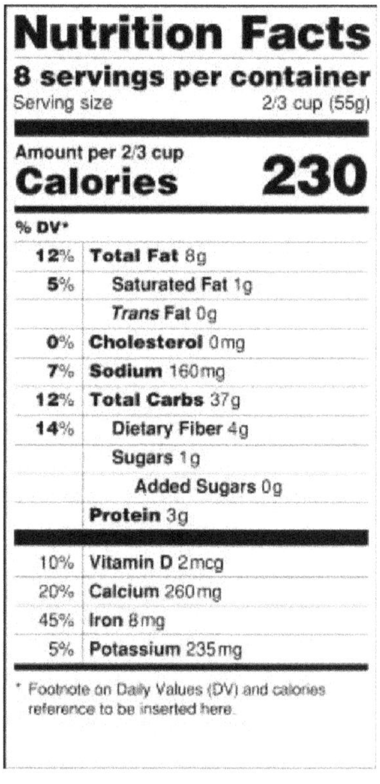

Recommendations

The government has made recommendations in regard to daily calorie intake and the amounts of carbohydrates, protein and fats in the diet. It also has recommendations for the amounts of the particular food groups: breads, meats, oils, fruits, and vegetables. Most individuals enjoy their freedom of choice and do not necessarily like to be told what to do. However, it may be helpful to keep in mind that the recommendations are based on what research has shown. Studies that have been done evaluate the effects of certain foods on our health and well-being. The daily USDA recommendations are 6–11 servings of

Nutrition Facts		
8 servings per container		
Serving size		2/3 cup (55g)
Amount per 2/3 cup		
Calories		**230**
% DV*		
12%	**Total Fat** 8g	
5%	Saturated Fat 1g	
	Trans Fat 0g	
0%	**Cholesterol** 0mg	
7%	**Sodium** 160mg	
12%	**Total Carbs** 37g	
14%	Dietary Fiber 4g	
	Sugars 1g	
	Added Sugars 0g	
	Protein 3g	
10%	Vitamin D 2mcg	
20%	Calcium 260mg	
45%	Iron 8mg	
5%	Potassium 235mg	

* Footnote on Daily Values (DV) and calories reference to be inserted here.

FIGURE 17.1   Food Label.

bread, cereal, rice, and pasta group; 3–5 servings of the vegetable group; 2–4 servings of the fruit group; 2–3 servings of the milk, cheese, and yogurt group; 2–3 servings of the meat, poultry, fish, dry beans, eggs, and nuts group; and sparing use of fats, oils, and sweets. The recommendations are detailed in full in Figure 17.1.

NEED TO KNOW

Sometimes the choice is not obvious. Say you are thirsty and stop at a convenience store to purchase a cold drink. You see the following choices in the cooler: Red Bull, Simply Orange, Gatorade, and POM juice. You would like to choose the drink with the least amount of added sugar. Which one do you chose?

  A. Red Bull: 27 grams of sugar (7 tsp)
  B. Simply Orange: 41 grams of sugar (10 tsp)
  C. Gatorade: 42 grams of sugar (10.5 tsp)
  D. POM: 62 grams of sugar (15.5 tsp)

It is best to read the nutritional label information on each to make an informed choice and not to follow your instinct.

References

1. https://www.fda.gov/food/ingredientspackaginglabeling/labelingnutrition/ucm436722.htm
2. Schulze, M. B., Manson, J. E., Ludwig, D. S., Colditz, G. A. et al. (2004). Sugar-sweetened beverages, weight gain, and incidence of type 2 diabetes in young and middle-aged women. *Journal of the American Medical Association, 292*(8), 927–934.
3. Palmer, J. R., Boggs, D. A., Krishnan, S., Hu, F. B. et al. (2008). Sugar-sweetened beverages and incidence of type 2 diabetes mellitus in African American women. *Archives of Internal Medicine, 168*(14), 1487–1492. doi:10.1001/archinte.168.14.1487
4. Löfvenborg, J. E., Andersson, T., Carlsson. P.-O. et al. (2016). Sweetened beverage intake and risk of latent autoimmune diabetes in adults and type 2 diabetes. *European Journal of Endocrinology, 175,* 605–614.
5. https://www.nhlbi.nih.gov/health/educational/wecan/eat-right/distortion.htm

Resource

U.S. Food and Drug Administration—Site of the FDA to inform consumers the background of labeling and packaging of foods: www.fda.gov/food/ingredientspackaginglabeling

Figure Credit

Fig. 17.1: Source: https://commons.wikimedia.org/wiki/File:FDA_Nutrition_Facts_Label_2014.jpg.

18

Exercise

Objectives

- ▶ Basic understanding of the different types of exercises
- ▶ Understanding of targeted heart rate
- ▶ Review of current recommendations
- ▶ Discussion of the benefits of exercise

Exercise

Exercise can be described as physical activity for the purpose of improving or sustaining one's health. There are four main types of exercise: endurance, strength, balance, and flexibility. Each type has different benefits for improving one's health or fitness. A combination of the different types of exercise will provide individuals with the most health benefits. If the focus is entirely on strength, deficits in flexibility may prove problematic. Similarly, balance improvements will likely require strength improvements.

Endurance

Endurance exercises are activities that focus on improving one's aerobic (oxygen-related) capacity. *Aerobic* exercises focus on improving the oxygen-carry capacity of the body. We obtain oxygen when we breathe; the oxygen enters red blood cells during an exchange of oxygen for carbon dioxide in the lungs. The heart then pumps the oxygenated blood throughout the body for use in all cells. Endurance exercise works to improve efficiency of the lungs and heart.

Beginning an endurance program is generally the hardest step. Some may have difficulty carving out time in a busy schedule, but it is the most important step to initiate a program. In most individuals, medical clearance is not required to initiate a program. There are certain patient demographics for whom it would be best to have physician clearance before beginning such a program.

The American College of Sports Medicine recommends people see their physician prior to starting an exercise program if two or more of the following apply to their situation: age greater than 35, high blood pressure, high cholesterol, diabetes, current or recent (within past 6 months) smoking, or a family history of heart disease before age 60. If unsure, it always best to consult first with a physician.

Heart rate (HR) is the speed of the heartbeat and reflects the number of heart contractions in 1 minute. It is usually expressed as beats per minute (bpm). You can take your HR by feeling for changes in pressure of the arteries (pulse). This is most commonly done at the level of the wrist. The number of pulsations are then counted over a 1-minute time period. You can also estimate your pulse by timing over a 30-second time period and then doubling the number. Recently, smart phones and exercise watches have incorporated technologies to take one's pulse.

The *maximum HR* is the maximum number of heart beats per minute during exercise. The formula to determine maximum HR is 220 minus the age of the individual. For example, the maximum HR in a 20-year-old individual is $220 - 20 = 200$ bpm and in a 60 year old is $220 - 60 = 160$ bpm. It is recommended not to exceed this value. Most aerobic or endurance exercise is performed at a level of 80% of the maximum HR. The *target HR* for a 20-year-old college student who wishes to exercise at the 80% level is 160 bpm. This is calculated by multiplying the individual's maximum HR, 200, by .80, or $200 \times .80 = 160$ bpm. This is the target HR for the student to maintain during the exercise routine that will result in improving his or her fitness.

The *resting HR* is defined as the number of bpm at rest. This number will vary significantly from patient to patient. Why the variation? One cause may be related to medications. Certain medications can either increase or decrease the HR. Similarly, caffeine can cause increases in the HR. Fitness is also a major determinant of resting HR; the fitter individuals are, the lower their resting HR will be.

The heart is a muscle, and muscles can improve their strength and size when they are challenged, such as when lifting weights. With regular fitness exercise, the heart gets more and more efficient, particularly at pumping blood. Blood is pumped out to the rest of the body. The amount of blood that is pumped out over a period of time is referred to as cardiac output. Cardiac output is the product of HR and stoke volume (the amount of blood that is pumped out with each heartbeat). Aerobic or endurance training will improve the stoke volume aspect of cardiac output. In response, since the heart is pumping out more blood with each beat, it can reduce the number of beats per minute and maintain its cardiac output.

Endurance exercises include running, cycling, and swimming, all of which can improve fitness in individuals. When the body is engaged in this type of exercise for a sustained period of time, endorphins are released. Endorphins are natural chemicals produced by the body that are similar to morphine. They can help ease pain and improve mood in those who exercise regularly, producing the "runner's high."

Strength

Strength training refers to exercises that improve muscle power and efficiency. Muscles work by contracting or shortening their length. They typically will cross a joint of the body and occasionally two joints. The muscle end is known as a tendon. The tendon will connect the end of the muscle to a bone. The contraction or shortening of the muscle will produce movement of the bone and joint. The muscle has one anatomic function; it can act as a flexor or an extensor. Flexors will flex the extremity, while extensors will act in an opposite direction to extend them. When the biceps contract, this results in flexion of the elbow; when the opposing muscle group, the triceps, contract, they extend the elbow.

There are different types of contractions a muscle may engage in. These contractions are known as isotonic, isometric, and isokinetic. The prefix translates to "equal."

Isotonic contractions maintain constant tension in the muscle as the muscle changes length. This can occur only when a muscle's maximal force of contraction exceeds the total load on the muscle.[1] Isotonic muscle contractions can be concentric or eccentric. Concentric contractions are when the muscle shortens. In contrast, eccentric contractions are when the muscle lengthens. An example of a concentric contraction is using a dumbbell to do a biceps curl; as the weight is lifted up, the biceps concentrically contracts, flexing the elbow and lifting the weight. As the weight is lowered, the biceps will contract eccentrically, slowly lowering the weight. If the biceps did not eccentrically contract, the weight would suddenly drop. Eccentric exercises are associated with greater strength gains.

Isometric contractions will generate force without changing the length of the muscle. This is typical of muscles found in the hands and forearm: The muscles do not change length, and joints are not moved, so force for grip is sufficient.[1] An example of this occurs when performing a chin-up. When a person holds his or her position at the top before beginning to lower, the muscles in this position are performing an isometric contraction—there is no movement, but they are active in maintaining a static position.

The third and final type of muscle contraction is an *isokinetic contraction*. This type of contraction is performed when the limb is in constant motion and variable resistance is applied. This type of exercise will engage in contracting the muscles with movement of a limb. An example of this muscle is when one uses a stationary cycle, maintaining it in a constant motion with the potential for variable resistance.

Muscles function to move our extremities. They are also responsible for controlling our core to help maintain our balance.

Balance

One may not necessarily think of improving balance as an exercise, but maintaining balance is crucial, especially as we age. Impaired balance in the elderly may result in a hip fracture, which can have devastating consequences. Balance is like any other skill one may learn: Use it or lose it. Specific exercises to safely challenge balance can improve both balance and coordination. These improvements can reduce risk of falls while serving to improve one's core strength.

Tai chi is an ancient Chinese discipline that focuses on the mind and body. The gentle movements emphasize certain postures and place additional mental focus on breathing and relaxation. The movements or sets of movements are typically practiced while standing. Studies have examined the potential positive effects of Tai chi. One study found that older people who took part in a 15-week Tai chi program reduced their risk of multiple falls by 47.5%.[2]

Another study showed that Tai chi movements to improve balance and strength among older people were effective. These improvements, particularly in strength, were preserved over a 6-month period in participants who did the Tai chi exercises.[3]

Flexibility

Another type of exercise is directed at improving flexibility. Flexibility exercises function to stretch muscles and their associated tendons. These exercises allow for improved movements as well as promote a maximal range of motion for joints. Improving one's flexibility is one of the first steps in addressing back pain. Low back pain is commonly seen in conjunction with hamstring contractures. The hamstrings are found in the posterior thigh region of the body. The muscles originate in the lower pelvic area and insert below the knees. The hamstrings function to flex the knees. The question is whether the hamstring tightness or inflexibility leads to low back pain or the low back pain plays a role in causing the hamstring muscles to become tight. It may be that certain painful positions of the back are improved with slight knee flexion, thereby promoting increased tightness in the hamstrings. Other muscles that develop tightness and inflexibilities are the neck muscles, shoulder muscles, and hip muscles. These inflexibilities can contribute to the cycle of increased pain and then increased inflexibilities leading to further increased pain, and so forth.

Flexibility exercises are most beneficial if done when the muscles are warm and not cold. Stretching a muscle will have the greatest benefit if done after the 3-mile run and not before the run. After the run the muscles are considered warmed up. One can also effectively stretch muscles by applying a moist heating pad to the muscle for 20 minutes prior to the stretching or also stretching after a warm shower or bath.

Recommendations

The U.S. government recommends adults get at least 2.5 hours of moderate-intensity aerobic exercise each week, or 1 hour and 15 minutes of vigorous-intensity activity, or a combination of both. It is also recommended that adults engage in muscle-strengthening activities twice per week. These recommendations are based on the findings of multiple research studies. Given the hectic pace of our lives today, it is important that one makes the time for exercise. Just knowing the recommendations affords no health benefits.

Benefits

The benefits of exercise are numerous. The benefits fall into four categories: enhancing function, maintaining reserve capacities, preventing disease, and ameliorating the effects of age and chronic disease.[4] Specifically, exercise has shown to do the following: reduce the risk of heart attack, stroke, breast cancer, colon cancer, prostate cancer, endometrial cancer, anxiety, depression, dementia, osteoporosis, and falls; elevate mood; increase intellectual functioning; improve self-esteem; control weight; decrease symptoms of Parkinson's disease; improve pain of fibromyalgia; and increase bone mass.[2-10] The benefits of exercise have been shown to improve one's morbidity and mortality in a number of physical, mental, and emotional domains.

NEED TO KNOW

For centuries, mankind has searched for the fountain of youth. It was searched for extensively by Ponce de León in the area that is now Florida. The fountain has never been found, although one may argue the benefits of exercise are in some way a fountain of youth.

Jack LaLanne was a true believer in the value and importance of exercise and fitness. He promoted healthy living on television and via his lifestyle. He completed extraordinary feats, which included the following:

At *age 45* he completed 1,000 pushups and 1,000 chin-ups in 1 hours and 22 minutes; at *age 60* he swam from Alcatraz Island to Fisherman's Wharf handcuffed, shackled, and towing a 1,000-pound boat; and at *age 70* he was handcuffed, shackled, and fighting strong winds and currents as he towed 70 boats with 70 people from the Queensway Bridge in Long Beach Harbor to the *Queen Mary*, a distance of 1½ miles. Sometimes things such as the fountain of youth can be hidden in plain sight.

References

1. Types of muscle contractions: Isotonic and isometric. (2015). Boundless Anatomy and Physiology. Retrieved from https://www.boundless.com/physiology/textbooks/ boundless-anatomy-and- physiology-textbook/muscle-tissue-9/control-of-muscle-tension-97/ types-of-muscle- contractions-isotonic-and-isometric-546-8434/
2. Wolf, S. L., Barnhart, H. X., Kutner, N. G., McNeely, E., Coogler, C., & Xu, T. (1996). Reducing frailty and falls in older persons: An investigation of tai chi and computerized balance training. *Journal of the American Geriatrics Society, 44*(5), 489–497.

3. Wolfson, L., Whipple, R., Derby, C., Judge, J., King, M., Amerman, P., Schmidt, J., & Smyers, D. (1996). Balance and strength training in older adults: Intervention gains and tai chi maintenance. *Journal of the American Geriatrics Society, 44*(5), 498–506.

4. Fentem, P. H. (1994). ABC of sports medicine: Benefits of exercise in health and disease. *BMJ, 308,* 1291.

5. Cruise, K. E., Bucks, R. S., Loftus, A. M., Newton, R. U., Pegoraro, R., & Thomas, M. G. (2011). Exercise and Parkinson's: Benefits for cognition and quality of life. *Acta Neurologica Scandinavica, 123, 13–19.* doi: 10.1111/j.1600-0404.2010.01338.x

6. Anthony, J. (1991). Psychologic aspects of exercise. *Clinics in Sports Medicine, 10*(1), 171–180.

7. Vainio, H., & Bianchini, F. (2002). *Weight control and physical activity* (Vol. 6). Lyon, France: International Agency for Research Cancer Press.

8. Patel, A. V., Rodriguez, C., Bernstein, L. et al. (2005). Obesity, recreational physical activity, and risk of pancreatic cancer in a large US cohort. *Cancer Epidemiology, Biomarkers and Prevention, 14,* 459–466.

9. Patel, A. V., Callel, E. E., Bernstein, L. et al. (2003). Recreational physical activity and risk of post-menopausal breast cancer in a large cohort of US women. *Cancer Causes and Control, 14,* 519–529.

Resources

Centers for Disease Control and Prevention—CDC sponsored site on the recommendations and different types of exercises with links to the proven health benefits: https://www.cdc.gov/physicalactivity/basics/adults/index.htm

Jack LaLanne—Website devoted to the "Godfather of Modern Fitness," this site reviews his basic principles and details the incredible feats he achieved throughout his life. Very inspiring site to promote the benefits of fitness: http://jacklalanne.com

19

Complementary and Alternative Medicine

Objectives

- ▸ Basic understanding of complementary medicine
- ▸ Basic understanding of alternative medicine
- ▸ Basic understanding of integrative medicine
- ▸ Review of the literature of complementary and alternative medicine treatments

Complementary Medicine

Complementary medicine refers to a group of therapeutic and diagnostic disciplines that exist largely outside the institutions where conventional health care is taught and provided.[1] Complementary medicine treatments can be used along with traditional medicine.

Alternative Medicine

Alternative medicine includes treatments that are used in place of conventional or traditional medicine. Currently, there is no standardized, national system for credentialing complementary health practitioners. State and local governments are responsible for deciding what credentials practitioners must have to work in their jurisdiction. Given the fact that each state will credential providers differently, there is tremendous variation in the disciplines from state to state.

This chapter will review a limited list of the more popular treatments; this is by no means a complete list. There are numerous complementary and alternative medical treatments available to consumers.

Acupuncture

Acupuncture has its roots in Eastern medicine and originated in China more than 2,000 years ago. It is based on the belief that a life force, or energy, known as "qi" flows through meridians in the body. The meridians are energy pathways, with each meridian corresponding to an organ or group of organs

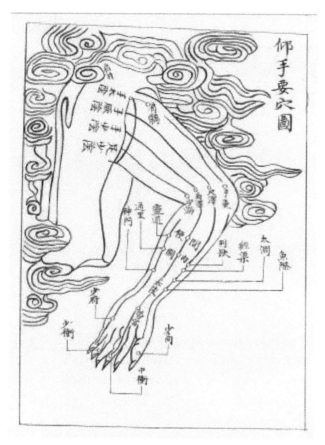

FIGURE 19.1 Acupuncture Meridians of the Arm published in 1742.

that govern particular bodily functions. Disease is believed to be an imbalance of qi, while a healthy state is believed to be in balance. Qi maintains the balance of yin and yang (which are opposites). Acupuncture involves inserting very small needles into the skin to stimulate the body's meridians to correct imbalances and to restore health.

In contrast, many Western practitioners view the acupuncture points as places to stimulate nerves, muscles, and connective tissue. Some believe that this stimulation boosts the body's natural painkillers and increases blood flow. How acupuncture works is not entirely clear. One possible explanation is that the needling process may produce a variety of effects in the body and the brain. Acupuncture has been demonstrated to enhance endogenous opiates such as dynorphin, endorphin, and encephalin and to release corticosteroids, relieving pain and enhancing the healing process.[2]

Research continues to be done on the effectiveness of acupuncture for a variety of conditions. Research has shown acupuncture to be effective in treating morning sickness associated with pregnancy as well as in the treatment of postoperative pain following a cesarean section.[3] Limited evidence has shown that acupuncture is modestly effective for acute low back pain.[4] Acupuncture has also been shown to be beneficial in helping treat pain associated with peripheral neuropathy (nerve pain).[5]

Aromatherapy

According to the National Center for Complementary and Integrative Health, aromatherapy is the use of essential oils from plants (flowers, herbs, or trees) as therapy to improve physical, emotional, and spiritual well-being. Essential oils like those from Roman chamomile, geranium, lavender, or cedar wood are the basic materials of aromatherapy.

Essential oils used in aromatherapy are extracted from various parts of plants which undergo a distillation process. The highly concentrated oils are then inhaled or applied topically to the skin. The oils may be applied to the skin via massage.

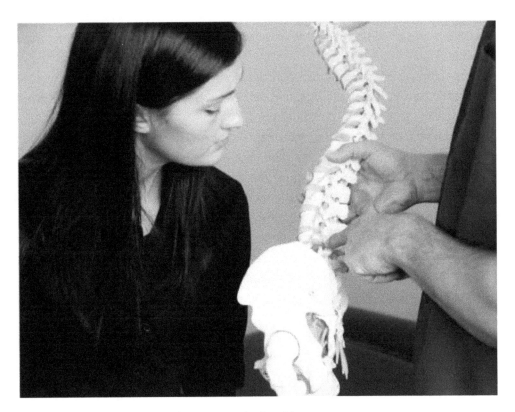

FIGURE 19.2   Chiropractors specialize in treating back problems.

Aromatherapy may work by stimulating the smell receptors in the nose and body. This activation sends information to the central nervous system. The limbic system, which helps control emotions, is thought to be stimulated. This type of therapy may produce an environment or sensation that can lead to relaxation, reduction of stress, and additional positive health effects. Studies supporting the use of aromatherapy are limited. Research has shown that aromatherapy massage may have potential to be used as an effective therapeutic option for the relief of depressive symptoms in a wide variety of subjects.[6] Aromatherapy has also been used to treat the pain associated with cancer, although there is a lack of evidence to support the clinical effectiveness of aromatherapy massage for symptom relief in people with cancer.[7] In addition, aromatherapy and massage have been used to treat the behavioral issues associated with dementia, but at this time the benefits are equivocal.[8]

Chiropractic

Chiropractors use hands-on spinal manipulation and other alternative treatments, to properly align the body's musculoskeletal structure, particularly the spine. This technique, is believed to enable the body to heal itself without the need of surgery or medications.

Manipulation is used to restore mobility to joints restricted by tissue injury caused by a traumatic event, such as falling, or repetitive stress, such as sitting without proper back support.

Chiropractic manipulation and treatments are primarily used as a pain relief alternative for muscles, joints, bones, and connective tissue such as cartilage, ligaments, and tendons. It may sometimes be used in conjunction with conventional medical treatment. Chiropractors treat a variety of clinical conditions, including back and neck pain, whiplash and soft tissue injuries, and chronic spine issues.

Training to become a chiropractor generally takes about 7 to 8 years of education. Training requires completion of an undergraduate education at a college or university, typically taking 4 years. Chiropractic students then complete 3 to 5 years at a chiropractic school to earn their degree, denoted as DC. Following graduation, they will enter into a 1-year clinical internship. In the United States the Council on Chiropractic Education (CCE) accredits chiropractic programs and institutions. Currently, 18 U.S. programs are accredited by the CCE. Twelve programs outside the United States are also accredited through affiliated chiropractic education councils.

Herbal Medicine

Products made from botanicals, or plants, which are used to treat diseases or maintain health are called herbal products. When a product made entirely from plants is used solely for internal purposes, it is then known as an herbal supplement. Herbal supplements may contain entire plants or plant parts. Herbal supplements come in all forms: dried, chopped, powdered, capsule, and liquid.

Cranberries have been studied in regard to their potential health benefits. Research has focused on their use in preventing urinary tract infections. The results have been mixed, but it does appear that their effectiveness may be similar to antibiotics in preventing urinary tract infections, and they may work most effectively in preventing recurrent urinary tract infections in women.[9] Cranberry research has also focused on its role in maintaining dental health. Research suggests that cranberries may be effective in reducing dental caries and gingivitis.[10]

Garlic has long been portrayed by Hollywood as a potential deterrent against vampires. Does garlic provide effective health benefits? Research has shown that garlic supplementation reduced blood pressure by 7–16 mm Hg, and it also reduced total cholesterol by 7.4–29.8 mg/dL.[11] The findings are beneficial for reducing the risks of both heart attack and stroke.

The potential health benefits of ginger have also been touted. Ginger has been shown to be helpful in reducing high cholesterol, high blood glucoses, and inflammation.[12]

Studies suggest that the short-term use of ginger can safely improve pregnancy-related nausea and vomiting.[13]

Green tea has been used for centuries for medicinal purposes. The tea is rich in catechins. The health benefits of teas are related to these catechins. The inhibitory activities of tea catechins against carcinogenesis and cancer cell growth have been demonstrated in a large number of laboratory studies.[14] The results have not been as dramatic in clinical studies, but benefits have been shown. A meta-analysis looking at the effects of green tea on prostate cancer incidence showed a reduction of prostate cancer risk with consumption of seven or more cups per day of green tea.[15] Green tea was also studied in regard to risk of endometrial cancer, and results indicate that green tea, but not black tea, may be related to a reduction of endometrial cancer risk.[16]

Massage therapists use their fingers, hands, forearms, and elbows to manipulate the muscles and other soft tissues of the body. The different types are related to variations in different techniques used and include Swedish massage, deep tissue massage, and sports-directed massage.

In Swedish massage the focus is general, and the therapist may use long strokes, kneading, deep circular movements, vibration, and tapping. With a deep-tissue massage, the focus is more targeted, as therapists work on specific areas of concern or pain. These areas may have muscle knots, or places of tissue restriction. Sports-directed massage focuses on a specific area of concern and is directed at trying to massage swelling out of the limb, with techniques being directed toward the trunk.

Swedish massage for a total of 1 hour a week has been shown to improve resting blood pressure, heart rate, and inflammatory markers in hypertensive (high blood pressure) women.[17] Massage has also been studied in regard to its effects on preterm infants. Most studies reported that the administration of various forms of therapeutic massage exerted a beneficial effect on factors related to the growth of preterm infants. Specific benefits of massage therapy when administered to hospitalized preterm infants included better neurodevelopment, a positive effect on brain development, a reduced risk of neonatal sepsis, a reduced length of hospital stay, and reduced neonatal stress.[18]

Spiritual wellness is a personal matter involving values and beliefs that provide one with a greater purpose or existence in life. While different individuals may have different views of what spiritualism is, it is generally considered to be the search for meaning and purpose in human existence, leading one to strive for a state of harmony with oneself and others while working to balance inner needs with the rest of the world.

Aspects of spiritual wellness may include hope, love, and prayer. Hope is a positive attitude in the face of a trying or difficult situation. The power of hope is an important component in the recovery from a challenging medical diagnosis or problem. Love and family support are equally important attributes. Studies of children with chronic illness have shown that love and support of family results in better health outcomes.[19]

Prayer is the act of putting oneself in the presence of a higher power. Both individual and group prayer have been used throughout the ages and in multiple cultures. In a 1996 poll, one half of doctors reported that they believe prayer helps patients, and 67% reported praying for a patient. Researchers have also studied the power of prayer in medicine. A landmark study was done in San Francisco in 1988, in which a group of intensive care unit patients were prayed for and their outcomes compared to another group of patients. The prayer group of patients required less ventilatory assistance, antibiotics, and diuretics compared to the control group.[20]

Yoga has historical origins in ancient Indian philosophy. It emphasizes a focus on both mind and body. Yoga will combine physical postures along with breathing techniques, meditation, and relaxation. Yoga is classified as a low-impact activity and is generally safe for healthy people. Individuals with certain back problems may need to avoid certain poses to avoid putting additional stress on the back. Additionally, women who are pregnant should modify or avoid some yoga poses.

Current research suggests that a carefully adapted set of yoga poses may reduce lower back pain and improve function.[4] Other studies also suggest that practicing yoga may have beneficial effects on psychiatric and medical conditions. These include pregnancy, prenatal and postpartum depression, stress, post-traumatic stress disorder (PTSD), anxiety, and pain syndromes including arthritis and headaches.[21]

There are many training programs for yoga teachers throughout the country. These programs range from a few days to more than 2 years. Standards for teacher training and certification differ, depending on the particular style of yoga. There are organizations that register yoga teachers and training programs that have complied with a certain curriculum and educational standards. For example, the nonprofit Yoga Alliance requires at least 200 hours of training, with a specified number of hours in areas including techniques, teaching methodology, anatomy, physiology, and philosophy. The International Association of Yoga Therapists is developing standards for yoga therapy training to ensure better standards for consumers.

NEED TO KNOW

Magnets as a cure for a number of problems are often advertised on late-night television or in full-page magazine articles. They are marketed for many different types of pain, including foot and back pain from conditions such as arthritis and fibromyalgia. Various products with magnets in them include shoe insoles, bracelets and other jewelry, mattress pads, and bandages. Many studies have looked at the claims, with mixed results. However, many studies have not been of high quality, had a small number of subjects, or were too brief or not properly controlled. The majority of trials have found no effect on pain.[22-27]

References

1. Álvarez, M. J., Fernández, D., Gómez-Salgado, J., Rodríguez-González, D., Rosón, M., & Lapeña, S. (2017). The effects of massage therapy in hospitalized preterm neonates: A systematic review. *International Journal of Nursing Studies, 69*, 119–136. doi:10.1016/j.ijnurstu.2017.02.009

2. Bodet, C., Grenier, D., Chandad, F., Ofek, I., Steinberg, D., & Weiss, E. I. (2008). Potential oral health benefits of cranberry. *Critical Reviews in Food Science and Nutrition, 48*(7), 672–680. doi: 10.1080/10408390701636211

3. Byrd, R. C. (1988). Positive therapeutic effects of intercessory prayer in a coronary care unit population. *Southern Medical Journal, 81*(7), 826–829.

4. Chou, R., Deyo, R., Friedly, J., Skelly, A. et al. (2017). Nonpharmacologic therapies for low back pain: A systematic review for an American College of Physicians clinical practice guideline. *Annals of Internal Medicine, 166*(7), 493–505. doi:10.7326/M16-2459

5. Dimitrova, A., Murchison, C., & Oken, B. (2012). Acupuncture for the treatment of peripheral neuropathy: A systematic review and meta-analysis. *Current Opinion in Obstetrics & Gynecology, 24*(2), 65–71. doi: 10.1097/GCO.0b013e32834fead1

6. Dimitrova, A., Murchison, C., & Oken, B. (2017). Acupuncture for the treatment of peripheral neuropathy: A systematic review and meta-analysis. *Journal of Alternative and Complementary Medicine, 23*(3), 164–179. doi: 10.1089/acm.2016.0155

7. Eccles, N. K. (2005). A critical review of randomized controlled trials of static magnets for pain relief. *Journal of Alternative and Complementary Medicine, 11*(3), 495–509.

8. Field, T. (2016). Yoga research review. *Complementary Therapies in Clinical Practice, 24*, 145–161. doi: 10.1016/j.ctcp.2016.06.005

9. Forrester, L. T., Maayan, N., Orrell, M., Spector, A. E., Buchan, L. D., & Soares-Weiser, K. (2014). Aromatherapy for dementia. *Cochrane Database of Systematic Reviews, 2*, CD003150. doi:10.1002/14651858. CD003150.pub2

10. Guo, Y., Zhi, F., Chen, P., Zhao, K., Xiang, H., Mao, Q., Wang, X., & Zhang, X. (2017). Green tea and the risk of prostate cancer: A systematic review and meta-analysis. *Medicine, 96*(13), e6426.

11. Jepson, R. G., Williams, G., & Craig, J. C. (2012). Cranberries for preventing urinary tract infections. *Cochrane Database of Systematic Reviews, 10*, CD001321. doi:10.1002/14651858.CD001321.pub5

12. Khoromi, S., Blackman, M. R., Kingman, A. et al. (2007). Low intensity permanent magnets in the treatment of chronic lumbar radicular pain. *Journal of Pain and Symptom Management, 34*(4), 434–445.

13. McParlin, C., O'Donnell, A., Robson, S. C., Beyer, F. et al. (2016). Treatments for hyperemesis gravidarum and nausea and vomiting in pregnancy: A systematic review. *Journal of the American Medical Association, 316*(13), 1392–1401. doi:10.1001/jama.2016.14337

14. Perrin, J. M., & MacLean, W. E., Jr. (1988). Children with chronic illness: The prevention of dysfunction. *Pediatric Clinics of North America, 35*(6), 1325–1337.

15. Pittler, M. H., Brown, E. M., & Ernst, E. (2007). Static magnets for reducing pain: Systematic review and meta-analysis of randomized trials. *Canadian Medical Association Journal, 177*(7), 736–742.

16. Richmond, S. J., Brown, S. R., Campion, P. D. et al. (2009). Therapeutic effects of magnetic and copper bracelets in osteoarthritis: A randomised placebo-controlled crossover trial. *Complementary Therapies in Medicine, 17*(5–6), 249–256.

17. Rumbaut, R. E., & Mirkovic, D. (2008). Magnetic therapy for edema in inflammation: A physiological assessment. *American Journal of Physiology. Heart and Circulatory Physiology, 294*(1), H19–H20.

18. Sánchez-Vidaña, D. I., Ngai, S. P., He, W., Chow, J. K., Lau, B. W., & Tsang, H. W. (2017). The effectiveness of aromatherapy for depressive symptoms: A systematic review. *Evidence-Based Complementary and Alternative Medicine, 2017.* doi: 10.1155/2017/5869315

19. Shin, E. S., Seo, K. H., Lee, S. H., Jang, J. E., Jung, Y. M., Kim, M. J., & Yeon, J. Y. (2016). Massage with or without aromatherapy for symptom relief in people with cancer. *Cochrane Database of Systematic Reviews, 6*, CD009873. doi:10.1002/14651858.CD009873.pub3

20. Supa'at, I., Zakaria, Z., Maskon, O., Aminuddin, A., & Nordin, N. A. (2013). Effects of Swedish massage therapy on blood pressure, heart rate, and inflammatory markers in hypertensive women. *Evidence-Based Complementary and Alternative Medicine, 2013*, 171852. doi: 10.1155/2013/171852.

21. Vallbona, C., & Richards, T. (1999). Evolution of magnetic therapy from alternative to traditional medicine. *Physical Medicine and Rehabilitation Clinics of North America, 10*(3), 729–754.

22. Varshney, R., & Budoff, M. J. (2016). Garlic and heart disease. *Journal of Nutrition, 146*(2), 416S–421S. doi:10.3945/jn.114.202333

23. Wang, J., Ke, W., Bao, R., Hu, X., & Chen, F. (2017). Beneficial effects of ginger Zingiber officinale Roscoe on obesity and metabolic syndrome: A review. *Annals of the New York Academy of Sciences, 1398*(1), 83–98. doi:10.1111/nyas.13375

24. Yang, C. S., & Wang, H. (2016). Cancer preventive activities of tea catechins. *Molecules, 21*(12), E1679.

25. Zhou, Q., Li, H., Zhou, J. G., Ma, Y., Wu, T., & Ma, H. (2016). Green tea, black tea consumption and risk of endometrial cancer: A systematic review and meta-analysis. *Archives of Gynecology and Obstetrics, 293*(1), 143–155. doi: 10.1007/s00404-015-3811-1

26. Zollman, C., & Vickers, A. (1999). What is complementary medicine? *BMJ, 319*(7211), 693–696. Patil, S., Sen, S., Bral, M., Reddy, S. et al. (2016). The role of acupuncture in pain management. *Current Pain and Headache Reports, 20*(4), 22. doi: 10.1007/s11916-016-0552-1

Resources

Council on Chiropractic Education—: National agency that promotes and oversees chiropractic education including accreditation of schools and training programs: http://cce-usa.org/

National Center for Complementary and Integrative Health—NIH sponsored sites that provides answers to all topics A-Z in complementary medicine, consumer friendly site: https://nccih.nih.gov/

Figure Credits

Fig. 19.1: Copyright © Wellcome Images (CC by 4.0) at https://commons.wikimedia.org/wiki/File:Acupuncture_points_and_meridians._The_arm._Wellcome_L0035005.jpg.

Fig. 19.2: Copyright © Chiropractic Offices of Dr. T (CC by 3.0) at https://commons.wikimedia.org/wiki/File:Spinal_Decompression_Chiropractor_La_Jolla_Ca_-_panoramio.jpg.

20

Strength and Conditioning Coach

Objectives

- ▶ Familiarization with a strength and conditioning coach
- ▶ Understand a strength and conditioning coach's approach to training
- ▶ Review of the approach and emphasis in regard to strength and conditioning

Strength and Conditioning Coach

The strength and conditioning coach is a relatively new position, created in the 1970s by collegiate athletic programs. This discipline has continued to grow and evolve and is now an essential part of collegiate athletics. Its influence can also be seen in the private sector. The strength and conditioning coach's role has grown from being "the biggest guy in the gym," who advised and inspired

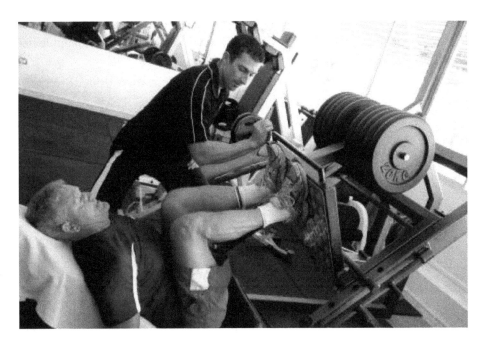

FIGURE 20.1   Personal trainer working with client.

other workout partners, to a profession that seeks to train clients in programs to enhance their health.

The collegiate emphasis of this position created the Collegiate Strength and Conditioning Coaches association (CSCCa), which is the main certifying organization of collegiate strength and conditioning coaches. The other national organization is the National Strength and Conditioning Association (NSCA), which is the world's leading membership organization. It oversees elite strength coaches, personal trainers, and dedicated researchers and educators. Both organizations offer certifications.

The CSCCa offers two levels of certification: the Strength and Conditioning Coach Certified and the Master Strength & Conditioning Coach. The certification process is a comprehensive one. To achieve certification, one must be a currently practicing, full-time strength and conditioning coach on the collegiate or professional level or a student preparing become a full-time strength coach on this level. The candidate must then complete a practical portion consisting of a 640-hour internship with a CSCCa-approved mentor. Prior to the oral examination portion, the candidate must write a comprehensive physical development program.

The candidate's written physical development program will be graded and evaluated by a panel of master strength and conditioning coaches. Then the candidate will need to successfully demonstrate lifting techniques and address potential modifications of the lifts for potential injuries. This is followed by a 350-question examination emphasizing the following subjects: muscle physiology, biomechanical concepts, aerobic and anaerobic exercise prescription, program design and periodization, free weight/machines/high-intensity training and techniques, nutrition/supplementation, and body composition/weight management.

The NSCA offers four credentialing programs: the Certified Strength and Conditioning Specialist (CSCS®), Certified Special Population Specialist (CSPS®), NSCA-Certified Personal Trainer (NSCA-CPT®), and Tactical Strength and Conditioning Facilitator (TSAC-F®).

The CSCS® is certification for professionals who design and implement strength training and conditioning programs for athletes in a team setting. The CSPS® is for fitness professionals who use an individualized approach to assess, motivate, educate, and train special population clients of all ages regarding their health and fitness needs, preventively and in collaboration with health care professionals. The NSCA-CPT® is for professional trainers who work with both active and sedentary clients in one-on-one situations. The TSAC-F® certification is for professionals looking to apply scientific knowledge to physically train military, fire and rescue, law enforcement, protective services, and other emergency personnel to improve performance, promote wellness, and decrease injury risk.

The certifications are helpful for consumers knowing that their trainers or coaches have attained appropriate knowledge and skills.

Training Philosophy

The training philosophy can vary some from coach to coach or trainer to trainer. Certain fundamentals are core to any training program. Full-service programs focusing on all assets of athletic development: addressing strength, power, speed, agility, conditioning, flexibility, recovery, nutrition, and injury prevention. Periodization of power development, strength, speed, agility, and conditioning programs all need to be tailored to the needs of the individual athlete for different micro-cycles of training. These parameters will change in response to the progress of the athlete/client. The concepts of injury preventatives, flexibility, recovery, and nutrition are emphasized on a constant basis and incorporated into all training workouts and programs.

High-Level Atmosphere

Coaches and trainers may display an intense environment with training. The outcomes will be improved when energy and excitement are incorporated into each training session. Competition is believed to breed success and may be creatively incorporated in each training cycle. Competing against teammates can inspire better outcomes; for clients, competing against previously set goals will allow appropriate future ones. Competitive environments are believed to build accountability and enhanced competitive drive.

Sport Science Monitoring

Technology has advanced significantly in the science of sport monitoring. Watches and phones can now track distance traveled, speed, heart rate, and calories burned and store workouts. The results can be used to compare results from previous workouts to set new goals. The technologies for collegiate and professional athletes can further evaluate recovery rates, effort, and body composition. Sleep tracking has also been an additional area of evaluation and point of emphasis. This information allows for objective tracking of gains and appropriate goal setting.

When muscles are challenged with weight, they will usually respond to the challenge by improving their power via changes in size. Strength training can utilize a free weight or a machine-based system. Free weights require balance of the weight to successfully lift. The machine-based program may allow for more isolated training of certain muscles and muscle groups.

Exercises that place an emphasis on total body athletic movements are denoted as the big three: clean, squat, and bench. Auxiliary lifts focusing on single leg/arm movements are utilized to strengthen bodily imbalances of musculature and increase strength balances through a full range of motion and increased flexibility.

An approach to conditioning can involve a variety of training. One can take a velocity-based approach to conditioning. Training speeds and recovery times can be monitored and used to set goals. Sport-specific conditioning will focus on improvements in the aerobic and anaerobic systems, as necessary to the needs and similarities of each sport (e.g., a football play is about 3 seconds, while a hockey shift requires more aerobic base comparatively, as it lasts about 2 minutes). The focus will be on improving heart and lung capacity and efficiency.

Testing for improvements are an important aspect of training at any level. The results will show both the client and coach how successful the training program has been. For consumers looking to lose weight or change their body composition, the evaluation can be done with weekly weigh-ins or body fat monitoring. For those looking to improve their speed or strength, comparisons of previous times and amounts can be reviewed and compared. This monitoring can serve as an objective measure. The consumer is paying the professional for his or her time, but also the effort is being done with certain goals in mind. If the goals are not being met, changes to the program or the trainer should be considered.

Every training session should have a regenerative session at the end of it, regardless of whether it is a practice, strength, or conditioning session. The regeneration session can be thought of as a period, or the punctuation that ends all sentences. The regenerative sessions are necessary in order to recover and prepare for the next session. Sessions may include manual therapy, hot tubs, cold tubs, rollers, myofascial release, and massage.

Trainers should exhibit some degree of passion for what they do. Consumers should get a degree of satisfaction from working with trainers, knowing that the goals they set together will provide a strong degree of health benefits.

NEED TO KNOW

What is the best way to lift to improve your strength? How about the best way to increase one's bulk or for improved tone? See the chart below.

TABLE 20.1

	Power	Strength	Bulk	Tone
Percentage of maximum	90–100	80–90	60–80	40–60
Repetitions per set	1–3	5	10	>12
Number of sets	3–6	5	6	3
Rest period	5 minutes	4 minutes	1 minute	30 seconds

Resources

Collegiate Strength and Conditioning Coaches Association—Home page of the CSCCA, a national organization designed to represent and promote the collegiate strength and conditioning coach, also with information in regards to the certification process: http://cscca.org/

National Strength and Conditioning Association—Site of the NSCA devoted to advancing the strength and conditioning coach, with additional information regarding membership and certification: https://www.nsca.com/

Figure Credit

21

Athletic Training

Objectives

- ▸ Understanding of an athletic trainer and their role
- ▸ Knowledge of training and regulation requirements of an athletic trainer
- ▸ Review of the medical coverage provided by athletic trainers

Athletic Trainers

Athletic trainers (ATs) are allied health care professionals who collaborate with physicians and work primarily with professional sports, colleges, secondary schools, orthopedic and rehabilitation clinics, and wellness centers. ATs may work with people of all ages and skill levels. These athletes may include young children, college/professional athletes, or weekend warriors. ATs specialize in diagnosing and treating muscle and bone injuries. They are usually the initial responder to an athletic injury either in a practice or game scenario. They also work to prevent such injuries in athletes at all levels. The trainer is part of an athletic team and works with other health care professionals, coaches, parents, and athletic administrators. Other job responsibilities may include: creating and implementing athletic policy or establishing athletic protocols for injuries. ATs may work to develop guidelines specifically for concussions.

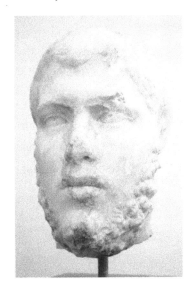

FIGURE 21.1 Head of a 3rd Century Kosmetes—athletic trainer; Archaelogical Museum, Athens Greece.

Work Environment

ATs tend to work in an educational setting. They may be employed by colleges, universities, or middle or high schools. Some trainers may work for professional sports teams, while others may be employed by a medical system, hospital, or physician's office. Irrespective of the setting, ATs work under the direction of a licensed physician. They work under a physician's supervising agreement. They will discuss specific injuries and treatment plans with the physician. Some trainers may meet with a team or consulting physician daily when a sport is in season.

Education

The Commission on Accreditation of Athletic Training Education (CAATE) accredits AT programs, including post professional and residency AT programs. ATs need to complete a CAATE-approved undergraduate program and obtain a bachelor's degree, or complete a CAATE-approved entry-level graduate athletic training education program. Master's degree programs are becoming more common. Athletic training degree classes may consist of a basic science portion that may include biology, chemistry, and physics. The clinical science portion may focus on anatomy, physiology, and nutrition. Additionally, degree programs will also emphasize a hands-on learning experience with a licensed trainer to serve as an instructor during a student's clinical rotations and clinical proficiencies. According to the U.S. Department of Labor, the job outlook for ATs is projected to grow 21% from 2014 to 2024. The department also notes that the median annual wage for ATs was $45,630 in May 2016.

Certification

Upon successful completion of the CAATE-approved program, graduates may sit for a national certification examination. The Board of Certification for the Athletic Trainer (BOC) is the national-level professional organization charged with certifying ATs and ensuring post certification requirements. The BOC offers the standard certification examination that most states use for licensing ATs. Certification requires graduating from a CAATE-accredited program and completing the BOC exam. Candidates must demonstrate proficiency in many competency areas. The specific areas are listed in Table 21.1. The competency areas cover a broad range of topics. The topics include the expected ones of pathology, assessment, and care for injuries and illness. Other topics include pharmacology, nutritional aspects of injury and illness, psychosocial intervention and referral, and health care administration.

ATs are licensed or otherwise regulated in 49 states and the District of Columbia. (Only California does not require a license.) The

TABLE 21.1   COMPETENCY AREAS FOR CAATE CERTIFICATION

Risk management and injury prevention

Pathology of injury and illness

Assessment and evaluation

Acute care of injury and illness

Pharmacology

Therapeutic modalities

Therapeutic exercise

General medical conditions and disabilities

Nutritional aspects of injury and illness

Psychosocial intervention and referral

Health care administration

Professional development and responsibilities

requirements vary by state. To maintain certification, ATs must adhere to the BOC Standards of Practice and Disciplinary Process and take continuing education courses.

Duties

ATs provide appropriate medical coverage. This not only involves monitoring and basic emergency care during sports participation, it also encompasses the provision of many other health care services for the student–athlete. (They are not just the people who run out on the field with a fanny pack and towel.) While emergency medical care and event coverage are critical, appropriate medical coverage also includes activities of ongoing daily health care of the student–athlete. ATs also will determine athletes' readiness to participate, in conjunction with the team physician. ATs will be involved in preparticipation evaluation and postinjury/illness return. They will work risk management and injury prevention for the athletes. ATs will also be paramount in the recognition, evaluation, and immediate treatment of athletic injuries/illnesses as well as the rehabilitation and reconditioning of athletic injuries. They may be the first to recognize an athlete's psychosocial issue and initiate an appropriate referral. They may also perform administrative tasks, such as keeping records and writing reports on injuries and treatment programs. They serve as the critical communication link between the athlete and coaching staff in regard to the injury and expected return-to-play plan.

Specifically, ATs work with athletes in sport-specific or functional exercises. They may also treat the athlete with specific modalities. The modalities (therapeutic agents) may be thermal, such as heat packs and ice, electrical, such as electrical stimulation, or therapeutic ultrasound. The trainer is also knowledgeable in the fit and application of braces and splints used for injury treatment and recovery. The trainer will set up a treatment schedule for the athletes. The treatment frequency will depend on the specific injury. The trainer may develop a close relationship to the athlete as they help them recover and rehabilitate. The AT serves an important role for the team and is integral to the athletes' and team's success.

NEED TO KNOW

When to use ice and when to use heat? Ice is used to decrease inflammation and is best used immediately after an injury or contest. The classic example of this is that the starting pitcher in baseball is immediately given an ice pack to place on his pitching arm after finishing the game. Ice is to be used within the first 72 hours of an injury. Ice can also be used to treat a muscle cramp or spasm. When applied to the offending muscle, it will cool the muscle spindles and allow for the muscle to relax and stop cramping. Heat is the modality of choice to increase blood flow to an area. It is best used after the initial 72 hours following an injury; then it can promote increased blood flow to the site of the injury and help promote healing and recovery.

Resources

Bureau of Labor Statistics—Site that details and overview of the profession, education, environment, pay and additional details of the athletic training profession: https://www.bls.gov/ooh/healthcare/athletic-trainers.htm

Commission on Accreditation of Athletic Training Education—Home page of the commission which accredits athletic training programs: https://caate.net

National Athletic Trainers' Association—Webpage for professional membership association for certified athletic trainers, this site explains the training and qualifications of an athletic trainer: http://www.nata.org

Figure Credit

22

Physical Therapy

Objectives

> ▸ Understanding of a physical therapist and their roles
> ▸ Knowledge of training and regulation requirements of physical therapist

Physical Therapist

According to the American Physical Therapy Association (APTA), physical therapists (PTs) are highly educated and licensed health care professionals who can help patients reduce pain and improve or restore mobility—in many cases without expensive surgery and often reducing the need for long-term use of prescription medications and their side effects. PTs can help educate and manage a patient's medical condition. They work to restore function and promote long-term health benefits. PTs work with individuals to formulate a plan specific to the needs of the individual in order to restore function and alleviate pain.

Work Environment

PTs can work in a variety of different settings. They may be employed by an acute care hospital, rehabilitation hospital, or clinic. They can also work for a private clinic or be the owner of their own practice. Approximately 25% of outpatient clinics are owned by a PT. Additionally, PTs may be employed by schools, home health agencies, work-hardening programs, wellness programs, hospice programs, and nursing homes. State licensure is required in each state in which a PT practices.

Education

The degree in physical therapy is now an advanced degree. Most therapy programs require a bachelor's degree as well as classes in anatomy, physiology, chemistry, biology, and physics as prerequisites. The Commission on

Accreditation in Physical Therapy Education (CAPTE) is an accrediting agency that grants accreditation status to training programs for PTs and physical therapist assistants. It is nationally recognized by both the U.S. Department of Education and the Council for Higher Education Accreditation. According to the CAPTE, there are currently 236 accredited training programs for PTs and 351 accredited training programs for physical therapy assistants. The prospective physical therapy student will apply through the Physical Therapist Centralized Application Service.

The training programs offer a doctor of physical therapy (DPT) degree. The DPT program is usually 3 years in length. There are some programs that will admit college freshmen into a combined bachelor's degree/DPT program. Such a combined program is 6 to 7 years in length and allows students to graduate with both a bachelor's degree and DPT. PT training programs often include courses in biomechanics, anatomy, physiology, and neuroscience. PT students also complete at least 30 weeks of clinical work, during which they gain supervised experience in areas such as acute care, rehabilitation care, and musculoskeletal issues. After graduation, PTs may apply to and complete a clinical residency program. Residencies are typically 1 year in length and provide additional training and experience in specialty areas of care. Therapists who have completed a residency program may choose to specialize further by completing a fellowship in an advanced clinical area.

The APTA has established a goal that by 2020 all PTs will be trained at the DPT level. According to the U.S. Department of Labor, the job outlook for PTs is projected to grow 34% from 2014 to 2024. The department also notes that the median annual wage for PTs was $85,400 in May 2016.

Physical Therapy Assistants

Physical therapist assistants (PTAs) provide physical therapy services under the direction and supervision of a licensed PT. Much like PTs, these assistants help people of all ages with medical or health-related problems. They provide care that may include patient education and training programs for ambulation and balance. In addition, PTAs may educate patients in the use of assistive devices, including canes and crutches. The assistant may also apply physical agents and modalities, including heat, ultrasound, and electrical stimulation.

The PTA needs to have earned an associate's degree, which is typically 2 years in length, from an accredited PTA program at a technical or community college, college, or university. Upon completion of the degree, graduates must pass the national examination for licensing/certification/regulation. PTAs work under the direction of a PT. PTAs are licensed or certified in all 50 states.

According to the U.S. Department of Labor, the job outlook for PTAs is projected to grow 40% from 2014 to 2024. The department also notes that the median annual wage for PTAs was $56,610 in May 2016.

Licensure

There is no national licensure entity for PTs or PTAs. The licensure is handled by each individual state. The licensing requirements vary from state to state, but all include passing a national physical therapy examination. The examination is administered by the Federation of State Boards of Physical Therapy (FSBPT). The FSBPT administers the National Physical Therapy Examination (NPTE), an examination that every graduate of a PT or PTA education program must pass to become a licensed PT or licensed/certified PTA in the United States. The NPTE is a computer-administered examination allotting 5 hours for 250 multiple-choice questions for PT candidates and 4 hours for 200 multiple-choice questions for PTA candidates.

Continuing education is typically required for PTs and PTAs to keep their license. Licensure is required in each state in which a PT practices and must be renewed on a regular basis. The majority of states also require continuing education requirements be met for renewal. After gaining work experience, some therapists may choose to attain board certification specialist status. The American Board of Physical Therapy Specialties offers certification in nine clinical specialty areas. These include cardiovascular/pulmonary, clinical electrophysiology, geriatrics, neurology, oncology, orthopedics, pediatrics, sports, and women's health. Board specialist certification requires passing an exam and at least 2,000 hours of clinical work or completion of an APTA-accredited residency program in the specialty area.

Duties

The duties of PTs can vary greatly, depending on the location of their practice and types of patients that they treat. Generally, PTs are educated and trained in a variety of different techniques to care for their patients. The fundamental principle is to improve function by enhancing the patient's ability to move. Focus is placed on the functional movement of the patient and the use of various exercise principles to improve strength, restore function, and promote mobility. PTs can provide care to people of all ages who present with functional limitations related to back pain, sprains (ligament injuries), strains (muscle injuries), stroke, spinal cord injury, traumatic brain injury, and neuromuscular conditions.

A PT may work as part of a health care team, supervising PTAs and working alongside physicians, occupational therapists, speech–language pathologists, and physiatrists in the rehabilitation setting. In rehabilitation settings, PTs often work with patients who have suffered devastating neurological injuries. PTs will emphasize mobility and,

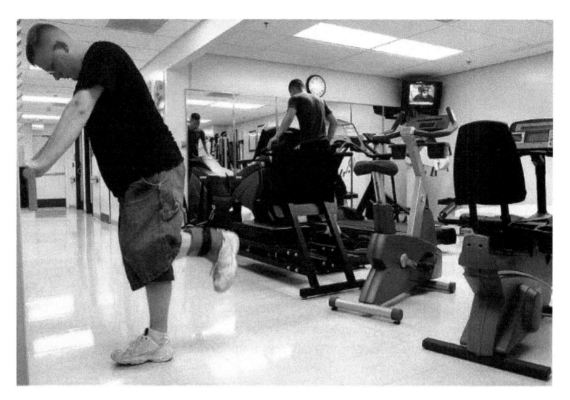

FIGURE 22.1   Exercising in a physical therapy gym.

depending on the patient's needs, may implement the use of canes, crutches, wheel-chairs, and walkers. They may devise a therapeutic treatment program that emphasizes the movements of joints, muscles, and other soft tissue to improve movement and decrease pain.

The specific work of PTs varies by type of patient. For example, a patient working to recover function lost after a spinal cord injury requires different care from a patient who is recovering from a sports injury or a stroke. Some PTs may specialize in one type of care, such as orthopedics, spinal cord injuries, or women's health issues. Some PTs may treat patients in the hospital setting (inpatient therapist), while other PTs work in an outpatient setting and treat patients after they are discharged from the hospital.

PTs develop individualized plans of care for patients after review of their medical history. This plan will need to outline patients' goals and the expected outcomes of the treatment program. The plan frequently needs to be submitted to the insurance company to permit continued care of services. The PT will need to continue to evaluate and record each patient's progress, modifying a plan of care and trying new treatments as needed. It is also important for the therapist to educate patients and their families about what to expect from the recovery process and how best to cope with future challenges. Home exercise programs are frequently established for patients after formal discharge from care.

Resources

American Board of Physical Therapy Specialties—link for the organization that develops standards for certification and subspecialty certifications and details these standards on this site: http://www.abpts.org/home.aspx

American Physical Therapy Association—Home page for the profession association that promotes advancement of physical therapy also includes a public section that describes the role of physical therapists in a variety of clinical capacities: https://www.apta.org

Bureau of Labor Statistics—Site that details and overview of the profession, education, environment, pay and additional details of the physical therapist profession: https://www.bls.gov/ooh/healthcare/physical-therapists.htm

Federation of State Boards of Physical Therapy—Site reviews the necessary requirements for the national examination and all the details associated with this examination: https://www.fsbpt.org/exam-candidates/nationalexam(npte).aspx; http://health.usnews.com/doctors

Figure Credit

Fig. 22.1: Source: https://commons.wikimedia.org/wiki/File:USMC-08184.jpg.

23

Occupational Therapy

Objectives

▸ Understanding of an occupational therapist and their roles
▸ Knowledge of training and regulation requirements of occupational therapists

Occupational Therapist

According to the American Occupational Therapy Association (AOTA), occupational therapists (OTs) are practitioners who enable people of all ages to live life to its fullest by helping them promote health, and prevent—or live better with—injury, illness, or disability. OTs can help to educate and manage a patient's medical condition. Much like physical therapists, OTs work toward restoring function and promoting long-term health benefits. OTs will work with individuals to formulate a plan specific to the needs of the individual in order to restore function and alleviate pain. Specifically, OTs help patients develop, recover, and improve the skills needed for daily living and working.

Work Environment

OTs can work in a variety of different settings. They may be employed by an acute care hospital, rehabilitation hospital, or clinic. According to the Bureau of Labor Statistics, about half of OTs work in occupational therapy offices or in hospitals. Others work in schools, nursing homes, and home health services. Occupational therapy is regulated in all 50 states. The regulation in some states may be licensure, while in others the regulations may be less rigorous. Regulation of OTs is done to reassure consumers of the training and necessary skill sets achieved and maintained by the therapist.

Education

The degree in occupational therapy is an advanced degree, with programs offering a master's or a doctoral degree. OT programs require a bachelor's degree as well as classes in anatomy, physiology, chemistry, biology, and physics as prerequisites. The AOTA is the agency that grants accreditation status to training programs for OTs and occupational therapist assistants. According to the AOTA, there are currently 175 accredited training programs offering the master's degree for occupational therapy and 16 accredited training programs offering the doctoral degree for occupational therapy. The prospective occupational therapy student will apply through the Occupational Therapy Centralized Application Service, which is a program of the AOTA. Much like with other centralized application services, the prospective student will submit one application to apply to multiple participating OT programs.

The training programs that offer a doctorate in occupational therapy (OTD) degree are typically 3 to 4 years in length. The training programs that offer a master's in occupational therapy (MOT) degree are typically 2 years in length. There are some programs that will admit college freshmen into a combined bachelor's degree/MOT program. Some combined programs are 5 years in length, allowing students to graduate with both a bachelor's degree and an MOT. OT training programs may include courses in neuroscience, musculoskeletal assessment, and occupational intervention. The training programs will emphasize fieldwork (hands-on experience) during the later years of the program.

According to the U.S. Department of Labor, the job outlook for OTs is projected to grow 27% from 2014 to 2024. The department also notes that the median annual wage for OTs was $81,910 in May 2016. OTs employed by nursing care facilities make a median income of $90, 380, and those employed by schools have a median income of $71,480.

Occupational Therapy Assistants

Occupational therapist assistants (OTAs) provide occupational therapy services under the direction and supervision of a licensed OT. Much like OTs, the OTAs help people of all ages with medical or health-related problems. They provide care that may include patient education and training programs for transfers and activities of daily living. In addition, OTAs may educate patients in the use of assistive devices, including long-handled shoe horns and adaptive eating utensils and plates. The assistant may also apply upper extremity splints to control tone and prevent hand and finger contractures.

The OTA needs to have completed an associate degree, which is typically 2 years in length, from an accredited OTA program at a technical or community college, college, or university. Upon completion of the degree, graduates must pass the national examination for licensing/certification/regulation. OTAs work under the direction of an OT. OTAs are licensed or certified in all 50 states. Each state has specific licensure requirements.

According to the U.S. Department of Labor, the job outlook for OTAs is projected to grow 40% from 2014 to 2024. The department also notes that the median annual wage for OTAs was $56,070 in May 2016, this is nearly identical to the wage of physical therapy assistants.

Licensure

There is no national licensure entity for OTs or OTAs. The licensure is handled by each individual state. The licensing requirements vary from state to state, but all include passing a national occupational therapy examination. The examination is administered by the National Board for Certification in Occupational Therapy (NBCOT). To sit for the NBCOT exam, candidates must have earned a degree from an accredited educational program and completed all fieldwork requirements. The NBCOT administers the occupational therapist registered (OTR) examination. The examination is 4 hours in length and consists of 170 multiple-choice questions and 3 clinical simulation test items. Passing the OTR examination is a requirement of every state in order to become a licensed occupational therapist in the United States. The AOTA also offers a number of board and specialty certifications for therapists who wish to demonstrate specialized knowledge in areas of practice, including pediatrics, mental health, and low vision.

OTAs will also need to complete training at an accredited program and successfully pass the NBCOT certified occupational therapy assistant (COTA®) exam to be licensed. Nearly all states require OTAs to be licensed or registered. Some states have additional requirements. OTAs must pass the NBCOT exam to use the title Certified Occupational Therapy Assistant.

Continuing education is typically required for OTs and OTAs to keep their license. Licensure is required in each state in which an OT practices and must be renewed on a regular basis. The majority of states also require continuing education requirements be met for renewal.

Duties

The duties of OTs can vary somewhat, depending on the location of their practice and the types of patients they treat. Generally, OTs work to maximize function of the patient. Whereas PTs are focused on mobility, OTs are focused on activities of daily living. Activities of daily living include dressing, feeding, and toileting. The fundamental principle is to improving the function of the patient. OTs' focus may be on the functional movement of the patient and the use of various exercise principles to improve strength, restore function, and promote independence. OTs can provide care to people of all ages who present with functional limitations related to upper extremity injuries, stroke, spinal cord injury, traumatic brain injury, and neuromuscular conditions.

Robert Louis Stevenson once said, "Life is not a matter of holding good cards, but of playing a poor hand well." This principle can be applied to patients treated by an OT. The patient has been dealt a new hand of cards in the game of life (e.g., suffering a stroke and not being able to move the right side of the body). In most cases one cannot change the hand one has been dealt, but the OT will work on helping individuals learn to play the new hand as best as they can, in terms of maximizing their new functional status.

The OT may work as part of a health care team, supervising OTAs and working alongside physicians, PTs, speech–language pathologists, and physiatrists in the rehabilitation setting, working to rehabilitate patients following a devastating neurologic injury. In this setting, OTs will emphasize upper extremity function. They may devise a therapeutic treatment program that emphasizes the movements of the shoulder, elbow and finger joints, muscles, and other soft tissue to improve movement and decrease pain.

The specific work of an OT varies by type of patient. For example, a patient working to recover function lost after a spinal cord injury requires different care from a student with developmental delay concerns. Some OTs may specialize in one type of care, such as pediatrics, spinal cord injuries, or return-to-work assessments. Some OTs may treat patients in the hospital setting (inpatient therapist), and the patients will need an outpatient therapist to treat them when they are discharged from the hospital.

The OT, much like the PT, will need to develop an individualized plan of care for the patient after reviewing their medical history. This plan will need to outline the patients' goals and the expected outcomes of the plan. The plan will then need to be submitted to the insurance company to permit continued care of services. The OT will need to continue to evaluate and record patients' progress, modifying a plan of care and trying new treatments as needed. It is also important for the therapist to educate patients and their families about what to expect from the recovery process and how best to cope with future challenges involved in establishing a home exercise program.

NEED TO KNOW

Adaptive equipment: OTs are the ones to see for adaptive equipment to improve function. They work with patients to maximize function. For example, patients with severe arthritic pain in the fingers may have difficulty cutting food, opening lids, and buttoning buttons. The OT can provide specific adaptive equipment to improve their function. Utensils may be modified or ordered with foam buildup requiring less force to hold them. A device also exists that allows buttons to be buttoned by placing a ring on the device through the buttonhole and around the button. These adaptive devices can save time and improve function.

Resources

American Occupational Therapy Association—Home page for the profession association that promotes advancement of occupational therapy with a section on careers and one for the public: https://www.aota.org

National Board for Certification in Occupational Therapy—Site reviews the necessary requirements for the national examination and all the details associated with this examination: http://www.nbcot.org/

Bureau of Labor Statistics—Site that details and overview of the profession, education, environment, pay and additional details of the occupational therapist profession: https://www.bls.gov/ooh/healthcare/occupational-therapists.htm

24

Speech–Language Pathologist

Objectives

- ▶ Understanding of a speech-language pathologist and their roles
- ▶ Knowledge of training and regulation requirements of a speech-language pathologist

Speech–Language Pathologist

According to the American Speech–Language Hearing Association (ASHA), speech–language pathologists (SLPs) work to prevent, assess, diagnose, and treat speech, language, social communication, cognitive-communication, and swallowing disorders in children and adults. Much like other therapists, SLPs work to restoring function and promoting long-term health benefits. SLPs will work with individuals to treat speech, communication, and swallowing disorders. They will also work to improve cognitive processing and memory in individuals.

Work Environment

SLPs work in a variety of different settings. They may be employed by an acute care hospital, rehabilitation hospital, or clinic. According to the Bureau of Labor Statistics, about 40% of SLPs work in schools. Almost all states require SLPs to be licensed. SLPs are regulated by each state in which they practice. The regulation requirements vary from state to state. Regulation of SLPs is done to reassure consumers of the training and necessary skill sets achieved and maintained by the therapist.

Education

The SLP is an advanced degree, with programs offering a master's degree. SLP therapy programs require a bachelor's degree as well as certain prerequisite classes in biology, human anatomy and physiology, linguistics, neuroscience, psychology, and physics (acoustics). The majority of individuals applying to graduate programs have a bachelor's degree in communication sciences disorders, but it is not required.

The Council on Academic Accreditation (CAA) is the agency that grants accreditation status to training programs for SLPs. According to the CAA, there are currently 249 accredited training programs offering the master's degree for speech–language pathology. The programs are monitored by the CAA on an annual basis to ensure compliance. The prospective SLP student will apply through the Council of Academic Programs in Communication Sciences and Disorders' Centralized Application Service. Much like other centralized application services, the prospective student will submit one application to apply to multiple participating SLP programs.

The training programs that offer a master's degree in speech–language pathology are typically 2 years in length. SLP training programs may include courses in audiology, aphasia, articulation, and augmentative communication. The training programs also emphasize clinical practice training in audiology, as well as communication and swallowing disorders, during the program.

According to the U.S. Department of Labor, the job outlook for SLPs is projected to grow 21% from 2014 to 2024. The department also notes that the median annual wage for SLPs was $74,680 in May 2016, with speech therapists employed by nursing care facilities making a median income of $92,220, and those employed by schools having a median income of $65,540.

Speech–Language Pathologist Assistants

Speech–language pathologist assistants (SLPAs) provide speech therapy services under the direction and supervision of a licensed SLP. SLPAs will assist the SLP with speech and language screenings. They will also follow the treatment plans as devised by the supervising SLP. They may also provide administrative support. Lastly, they may advocate for families through education and training programs.

The SLPA needs to have completed an associate's degree from a technical training program or a bachelor's degree in a speech–language pathology or communication disorders program. The candidate must also complete a minimum of 100 hours of supervised clinical work. Additionally, the SLPA must demonstrate competency of skills. Each state regulates SLPAs differently, with varying requirements. SLPAs work under the direction of an SLP. Some states do not recognize the use of SLPAs.

Licensure

There is no national licensure entity for SLPs. The licensure is handled by each individual state and varies from state to state. SLPs must pass an examination in order to obtain certification. According to the American Speech-Language-Hearing Association

(ASHA), the pass rate has been 84% to 90% over the past few years. The examination is known as the Praxis, and it is a national examination. Almost all states require SLPs to be licensed, and licensure requires at least a master's degree and supervised clinical experience.

SLPs can earn the Certificate of Clinical Competence in Speech–Language Pathology (CCC-SLP) offered by the ASHA. Certification satisfies some or all of the requirements for state licensure and may be required by some employers. In order to attain the CCC-SLP, one must pass the Praxis examination, complete an approved training program, and finish a clinical fellowship program.

The ASHA also recognizes a clinical doctoral degree in speech–language pathology (e.g., CScD, SLPD), an optional, post-entry-level clinical degree. The advanced degree will provide SLPs with the means for career advancement and professional development. This clinical degree is intended to prepare SLPs to become master clinicians, educators, administrators, or leaders in their specialty areas. The advanced degree typically takes 2 to 3 years in addition to the master's degree.

Another option recognized by the ASHA is the research doctoral degree. The research doctorate (PhD) in communication sciences and disorders prepares one for a faculty–researcher career to contribute to the body of knowledge that advances the science of the discipline. PhD graduates work in colleges and universities, research institutions, public or private agencies, industry, and so forth. The degree prepares one for future research emphasis. The degree may take an additional 3 to 5 years following the master's degree.

Continuing education is typically required for SLPs to keep their license. Licensure is required in each state in which an SLP practices and must be renewed on a regular basis. The majority of states also require that continuing education requirements be met for renewal.

Duties

The duties of SLPs can vary, depending on the location of their practice and types of patients that they treat. In an educational environment such as a school, SLPs will focus on communication. They will work with students to improve various speech disorders. They work to help students with language difficulties and may also focus efforts on enunciation. They may also perform similar tasks in an early intervention program.

The SLP who is employed in a rehabilitation setting may work with patients who have experienced an abrupt change in function following a stroke. Both the ability to swallow and speak may be affected following a stroke. Dysphagia is the term used to describe difficulty swallowing after a stroke. The SLP works with patients to improve their ability to swallow. The therapist may administer a swallowing study to assess the quality of a patient's ability to swallow.

The swallowing study may involve swallowing foods and liquids that are mixed with barium sulfate. Barium is a metallic compound that is visible on X-rays. The patient will swallow the food/liquids mixed with barium, and a fluoroscope will be used to evaluate the swallow, watching closely to make sure the food/liquid end up in the stomach and not the lungs. The therapist may try foods of different consistencies as well as liquids that may be thickened.

Additionally, speaking and communication may also be affected following a stroke. Aphasia (sometimes called dysphasia) is the term given when the clarity or enunciation of speech is affected. The stroke may leave a patient with weakness of the facial muscles. This weakness may make it difficult for the patient to control the muscles needed for clear speech. With the work of an SLP, these muscles can be strengthened. The therapist will work on a care plan to focus on strengthening the muscles. Communication and language can also be affected following a stroke. is the term given when one has difficulty finding the right words. Patients will aphasia may not be able to say the words that they are thinking; this can be a very frustrating problem for patients, as they are not able to express their wants and needs.

The SLP will work with patients to improve their aphasia, providing them with strategies to express themselves. In addition, augmentative communication devices also exist to overcome problems with communication. The SLP will be able to evaluate individuals for such devices and provide appropriate technology to allow for improved communication.

The SLP, much like the PT and OT, will need to develop an individualized plan of care for the patient after review of their medical history. This plan will need to outline each patient's goals and the expected outcomes of the plan. The plan will need to be submitted to the insurance company to permit continued care of services. The SLP will need to continue to evaluate and record each patient's progress, modifying a plan of care and trying new treatments as needed. It is also important for the therapist to educate patients and their families about what to expect from the recovery process and how best to cope with future challenges in establishing an appropriate home program.

Dysphagia (difficulty swallowing) can occur after a stroke. It is important to keep in mind that drinking liquids with dysphagia can lead to pneumonia. This specific type of pneumonia is known as aspiration pneumonia. Normally, when one swallows, the food/liquid will travel down the esophagus. A small flap of tissue called the epiglottis will then cover the bronchus (the tube that leads to the lungs). With the bronchus closed, the food/liquid will continue along the esophagus and into the stomach. Following a stroke, the epiglottis may not function properly to close the bronchus. This impaired function of the epiglottis can occur with dysphagia. If the epiglottis does not cover the bronchus, this can lead to food and liquid entering the lungs. The foreign material will lead to an infection and subsequent pneumonia. Liquids are more likely to enter the bronchus than food.

Resources

American Speech-Language-Hearing Association—Home page for the association which promotes the SLP profession with job descriptions and educational opportunities: http://www.asha.org

Council on Academic Accreditation—Site for SLP accreditation, outlines necessary steps: http://caa.asha.org

Bureau of Labor Statistics—Site that details and overview of the profession, education, environment, pay and additional details of the speech—language pathologist profession: https://www.bls.gov/ooh/healthcare/speech-language-pathologists.htm

Figure Credits

25

Physician Assistant

Physician Assistant

According to the American Academy of Physician Assistants, a physician assistant (PA) is nationally certified and state licensed to practice medicine as part of a physician-led team. PAs are educated at the graduate level and practice in nearly every medical specialty and setting.

There were concerns in the 1960s with the delivery of health care in the United States, as there was a shortage of primary care physicians. The 1965 White House Conference on Health was organized to address the health provider needs.[1] Out of this concern, the idea of other practitioners to provide care was conceived. The PA, nurse midwife, and nurse practitioner were proposed as solutions to the problem of health care delivery, particularly in rural areas.[2] Duke University School of Medicine was the first training program for PAs in the United States.

According to the Duke PA program website:

> *This idea led to the recruitment of four former navy corpsmen to compose the first class of Duke PA students. Three of these students completed the program and graduated in 1967.*

Notable changes have happened to PA training programs over the past 50 years. The profession, which started in part as a program for male veterans to transition into the civilian workforce is now predominately female and non-veteran.[4] The number of PA programs and students have continued to increase over the past 50 years. The Accreditation Review Commission on Education for the Physician Assistant is the accrediting agency that sets the standards for

PA education and evaluates PA training programs. There are currently 225 accredited PA training programs in the United States.

Work Environment

Because PAs need to be supervised by physicians, they tend to work in the same settings as physicians. They may be employed by a hospital or health care system or may work in a physician's private office or a group practice. According to the Bureau of Labor Statistics, about 57% of PAs work in physician's offices and 22% for a hospital or health care system. All states and the District of Columbia require PAs to be licensed. PAs are regulated by each state in which they practice. The regulation requirements vary from state to state. Regulation of physician assistants is done to reassure consumers of the training and necessary skill sets achieved and maintained by the PA.

Education

The degree to become a PA is an advanced degree, with programs offering a master's degree. PA programs require a bachelor's degree. GRE and MCAT scores are also important for applying. A fair number of candidates who apply for admission have a nursing, EMT, or other health care background as most programs may require prospective students to have about 3 years of health care experience, to ensure the candidate has some understanding of what a position in the medical field may entail. There are also certain prerequisite classes that are similar to medical school, including biology, anatomy and physiology, microbiology, chemistry, psychology, and statistics.

PA education programs are usually 26 months (3 academic years) of full-time study. The curriculum in year 1 may consist of didactics and labs as well as pathophysiology, pharmacology, physical exam and diagnosis, anatomy, procedures, and clinical decision making. In the second year, the curriculum will focus on clinical rotations in emergency medicine, family medicine, internal medicine, obstetrics/gynecology, pediatrics, psychiatry, and surgery.

The Accreditation Review Commission on Education for the Physician Assistant (ARC-PA) is the agency that grants accreditation status to training programs for PAs. According to the ARC-PA, there are currently 225 accredited training programs offering the master's degree for PAs. The programs are monitored by the ARC-PA on an annual basis to ensure compliance. The prospective PA student will apply to the Central Application Service for Physician Assistants, a service of the Physician Assistant Education Association (PAEA). This is the organization that represents PA educational programs nationwide. Much like other centralized application services, the prospective student will submit one application to apply to multiple participating PA training programs.

Admission into a PA school is competitive. Only 25% of applicants will be accepted to PA programs in any given year, according to the 29th PAEA Annual Report. Many top programs accept only about 2% of applicants, as noted on their websites.

According to the U.S. Department of Labor, the job outlook for PAs is projected to grow 30% from 2014 to 2024. The department also notes that the median annual wage for PAs was $101,480 in May 2016.

Licensure

The PA is nationally certified. To be eligible for certification, the PA must graduate from a program accredited by the ARC-PA and pass a national examination. Candidates must pass the Physician Assistant National Certifying Examination (PANCE) from the National Commission on Certification of Physician Assistants (NCCPA). The PANCE is a 5-hour computer-administered examination that consists of 300 multiple-choice questions administered in five blocks of 60 questions. According to the NCCPA, the pass rate for first-time takers is 96%. Any PA who passes the exam may use the credential Physician Assistant-Certified, or PA-C.

Continuing education is typically required for PAs to keep their certification. Licensure is required in each state in which a PA practices and must be renewed on a regular basis. PAs must complete 100 hours of continuing education every 2 years and a recertification examination is required every 10 years.

Duties

State laws require PAs to work under an agreement with a supervising physician. The PA would be able to work in a similar capacity as the supervising physician. For example, if the supervising physician is an internist, then the PA cannot assist in surgeries, and if the supervising physician is a surgeon, then the PA cannot serve as a neurological PA.

The physician does not need to be on-site at all times, but a level of collaboration is required. This oversight may have the physician also see patients the same day that they are treated by the PA. Another type of supervision may have the physician review and sign the medical record of every patient treated by the PA within 30 days of the treatment. In addition, the physician may have written protocols that specifically guide the actions of the PA. Working under the supervision of a physician, a PA can perform a number of tasks, as outlined in Table 25.1.

PAs are able to see patients independently and perform a history and physical examination of patients. After seeing a patient, PAs can diagnose and treat the illness. They also can order diagnostic tests, if needed, to determine a medical diagnosis or to follow an already diagnosed condition. They are also able to interpret the diagnostic tests and inform the patient of their results. PAs can also prescribe medications for the patient.

Some PAs are surgical in nature. They will perform a physical examination on a patient who is scheduled for surgery (pre-op patient). They may at that time order pre-op labs. These may include a CBC or electrolytes. In certain states, including California, if the supervising physician has delegated the PA authority to do so in writing. A PA may perform surgical procedures under local anesthesia without the personal presence of the supervising physician. A PA may perform surgical procedures requiring other forms of anesthesia only in the personal presence of the supervising physician. A PA may act as first or second assistant in surgery under the supervising physician.

TABLE 25.1   TASKS A PA CAN PERFORM

Take medical histories and perform physical examinations

Diagnose and treat illnesses

Order various diagnostic tests

Assist in surgery and outpatient procedures

Write prescriptions

NEED TO KNOW

PAs can also write prescriptions. They are currently able to write and prescribe schedule II substances in 49 states and the District of Columbia. Only the state of Kentucky does not allow PAs to prescribe Schedule II narcotics. This group of controlled substances includes Ritalin and Adderall, medications used for the treatment of ADD and ADHD.

References

1. Hooker, R. S., & Cawthon, E. A. (2015). The 1965 White House conference on health: Inspiring the physician assistant movement. *Journal of the American Academy of Physician Assistants, 28*(10), 46–51. doi:10.1097/01.JAA.0000471483.30681.78
2. Cawley, J. F., Cawthon, E., & Hooker, R. S. (2012). Origins of the physician assistant movement in the United States. *Journal of the American Academy of Physician Assistants, 25*(12), 36–40, 42.
3. https://cfm.duke.edu/about/history
4. Hooker, R. S., Robie, S. P., Coombs, J. M., & Cawley, J. F. (2013). The changing physician assistant profession: A gender shift. *Journal of the American Academy of Physician Assistants, 26*(9), 36–44.

Resources

Accreditation Review Commission on Education for the Physician Assistant—Site for the accrediting agency for PA training programs: http://www.arc-pa.org

American Academy of PAs—Homepage for the academy with information on the profession, educational opportunities and general news pertaining to PAs: https://www.aapa.org

National Commission on Certification of Physician Assistants—Webpage for certification testing outlining the necessary steps and testing information: http://www.nccpa.net/

Bureau of Labor Statistics—Site that details and overview of the profession, education, environment, pay and additional details of the physician assistant profession: https://www.bls.gov/ooh/healthcare/physician-assistants.htm

26

Psychologist

Objectives

- ▸ Understanding of a psychologist and their various roles
- ▸ Knowledge of training and regulation requirements of psychologists

Psychologist

According to the U.S. Department of Labor, psychologists study cognitive, emotional, and social processes and behavior by observing, interpreting, and recording how people relate to one another and their environments.

Work Environment

Some psychologists work independently conducting research, consulting with clients, or working with patients. Others work as a component of a health care team alongside physicians and social workers in medical or education settings. In education they work with students, teachers, and parents. According to the Bureau of Labor Statistics, about 33% of psychologists are self-employed, 25% work in elementary and secondary schools, and 10% are employed by the government. All states and the District of Columbia require practicing psychologists to be licensed. Psychologists are regulated by each state in which they practice. The regulation requirements vary from state to state. Regulation of psychologists is done to reassure consumers of the training and necessary skill sets achieved and maintained by the psychologist.

Education

The degree to become a psychologist is an advanced degree, with programs offering a doctoral degree. Some positions may require a master's degree, but the majority of training programs are at the doctoral level. Psychology training programs require a bachelor's degree. Undergraduate GPA and GRE scores are important in the application process. Some doctoral degree programs require applicants to have a master's degree in psychology; others will accept applicants with a bachelor's degree and a major in psychology. Research experience is highly desirable; some candidates may have 2 to 3 years of research experience or a master's degree in psychology.

Graduates with a master's degree in psychology can be employed as an industrial–organizational psychologist. If they work under the direction of a doctoral psychologist, they can work as psychological assistants in clinical, counseling, or research areas.

School psychologists will commonly earn the education specialist's degree (EdS). This specialized degree will require a minimum of 60 graduate semester credits and a 1,200-hour (30-week) supervised internship. Their education will include course work in both education and psychology.

Other educational options may include a PhD in psychology or a doctor of psychology degree (PsyD). A PhD in psychology is a research based degree that is obtained after writing a dissertation based on original research and defending the thesis with faculty. PhD programs typically include courses in statistics and experimental procedures.

The PsyD is a clinical degree and is often based on practical work and examinations rather than a dissertation. In clinical, counseling, school, or health service settings, students usually complete a 1-year internship as part of the doctoral program.

The Commission on Accreditation (CoA) is the agency that grants accreditation status to training programs for psychologists. It does not accredit undergraduate or master's level programs. According to the CoA, there are currently 394 accredited training programs offering the doctoral degree in clinical, counseling, and school psychology or a combination of these. The programs are monitored by the CoA on a regular basis to ensure compliance with educational and training aspects. The prospective student will need to apply to each specific graduate program; there is not a central application service. The process is similar to other professional schools. Following submission of the application, the applicant will hear a decision regarding an interview, typically in January. If granted an interview, the candidate will then meet the faculty at the program and wait on the school's decision to accept or reject him or her.

Admission into a doctoral psychology program is competitive. Only 24% of applicants were accepted into such programs, according to the American Psychological Association (APA). The acceptance rate was 60% for master's degree programs.

According to the U.S. Department of Labor, the job outlook for psychologists is projected to grow 19% from 2014 to 2024. The department also notes that the median annual wage for psychologists was $95,710 in May 2016.

Certification

Psychologists are nationally certified but are licensed by the particular state in which they practice. To be eligible for certification, psychologists must graduate from a program accredited by the CoA and must pass a national examination, the Examination for Professional Practice of Psychology (EPPP). The Association of State and Provincial Psychology Boards is the certifying agency for the EPPP. The EPPP is a computer-based examination that lasts 4 hours and 15 minutes and consists of 225 multiple-choice questions. According to the EPPP, the test covers eight content areas: biological bases of behavior; cognitive–affective bases of behavior; social and cultural bases of behavior; growth and life span development; assessment and diagnosis; treatment, intervention, prevention and supervision; research methods and statistics; and ethical, legal, and professional issues items. The APA reports the pass rate for first-time takers is 82%.

Psychologists may wish to specialize in a particular area. The American Board of Professional Psychology awards specialty certification in 15 areas of psychology, such as clinical health, couple and family, or rehabilitation. The American Board of Professional Neuropsychology also offers certification in neuropsychology. Board certification can demonstrate additional expertise in a specialty area. This additional certification is not required for most psychologists. Some hospitals and clinics may require additional certification.

Licensure

Licensing laws vary greatly by state. Most clinical and counseling psychologists will need to have earned a doctorate in psychology, completed an internship, and successfully completed 1 to 2 years of supervised professional experience, in addition to passing the EPPP. Continuing education is typically required by states for psychologists to keep their certification. Licensure is required in each state in which a psychologist practices and must be renewed on a regular basis.

Duties

The duties of a psychologist will depend on the specific type of training the psychologist has had as well as the environment of practice.

Clinical psychologists are trained to diagnose and treat mental, emotional, and behavioral disorders. They may help individuals with short-term personal issues, such as the loss of a spouse or loved one. They may also see patients on a long-term basis for chronic behavioral or mental issues. These may include depression or an anxiety disorder. They are trained in various techniques and counseling to effectively treat clients. They may also engage in diagnostic cognitive testing to better understand the issues and develop an approach to better treat and address the problems. They can provide services at the individual, family, or group level. They may run group sessions to help with treatment. They will design and provide patients with programs to work on behavior modification.

Neuropsychologists are a specialized subset of clinical psychologists who study the effects of brain injuries/disease, developmental disorders, or mental health conditions on behavior and thinking. They test patients with various cognitive conditions to determine the deficits on thinking. Neuropsychologists may perform extensive testing to better understand the effects of a concussion, stroke, or underlying ADHD. Understanding the problematic areas can then allow for an appropriate treatment plan.

Counseling psychologists help patients deal with and understand emotional and relationship problems. They may address problems that occur at home. Sometimes, they may need to address problems that occur secondary to stressors in the workplace. They will counsel patients to help manage their concerns. The management plan may include providing patients with visual imagery techniques, biofeedback, or a management plan.

Developmental psychologists will specifically address the psychological developmental progress. They can treat patients throughout the patients' lifetime. Developmental psychologists may be employed by a school. They may address student learning and behavioral problems, design and implement performance plans and evaluate performances, and counsel students and families. They also may consult with other school-based professionals to suggest improvements to teaching, learning, and administrative strategies. They will work with the student and the school to establish an appropriate treatment program. They may also work with elderly patients, focusing on problems associated with aging. These problems may include dementia or physical impairments that may affect individuals from an emotional standpoint.

Forensic psychologists work in the legal and criminal justice system. They can evaluate individuals to help judges or attorneys. They may also serve as an expert witness to provide testimony in such cases. They will specialize in civil or criminal casework.

Industrial–organizational psychologists apply their trained principles to the workplace. They work to help solve workplace problems or issues. They may be asked to specifically evaluate strategies to improve workplace morale, productivity, or workers' compensation issues. Their input may also be valued to address policy planning. Industrial–organizational psychologists may be master's-level psychologists.

Social psychologists help determine how behavior is influenced by community or social interactions. They may study and research these interactions and work on ways to identify and improve them.

Resources

American Board of Professional Psychology—Homepage of the professional psychology board which certifies psychologists: https://www.abpp.org

American Psychological Association—Website of the professional organization that represents psychologists in the US: http://www.apa.org/

Association of State and Provincial Psychology Boards—Site for certification and testing information and oversight of credentials: http://www.asppb.net

Bureau of Labor Statistics—Site that details and overview of the profession, education, environment, pay and additional details of the psychologist profession: https://www.bls.gov/ooh/life-physical-and-social-science/psychologists.htm

27

Mental Health Issues

Objective

> ▸ Basic understanding of some common mental health conditions and their appropriate management

Psychiatrist

Psychiatrists are physicians who complete a psychiatry residency and who specialize in the diagnosis and treatment of mental disorders. Psychiatrists will examine patients and determine whether the patient's symptoms are the result of a physical or mental issue, or combination of both. Diagnostic tests including laboratory tests may need to be done to evaluate the possibility of a metabolic cause. An example of this is mercury poisoning. Elevated levels of mercury in the body can cause a myriad of symptoms, including mood swings, irritability, insomnia (inability to sleep), and abnormal sensations, all of which can be seen with depression.

The psychiatrist may determine the best way to proceed for each patient. This may include prescribing a medication or referring to a psychologist for counseling.

Psychologist

A psychologist is usually an individual who has attained a doctorate and specializes in metal health issues. Psychologists are trained to diagnose and treat mental, emotional, and behavioral disorders.

They are trained in various techniques and counseling to effectively treat clients. They may also engage in diagnostic cognitive testing to better understand the issues in an approach to better treat and address the problems. They provide services at either the individual, family, or group level. They may also provide patients with programs to work on behavior modification. They do not prescribe medications.

Diagnostic and Statistical Manual of Mental Disorder

The *Diagnostic and Statistical Manual of Mental Disorder*, 5th Edition (DSM-V) is the standard used by mental health experts for the diagnosis of various mental health problems. It is compiled by the American Psychiatric Association, which states that the DSM-V is the product of more than 10 years of effort by hundreds of international experts in all aspects of mental health. The manual is updated regularly as more research is done to better understand mental disorders.

Neurodevelopmental Disorders

Neurodevelopmental disorders involve dysfunctions of the development of the central nervous system. These disorders mainly involve developmental brain dysfunction. This dysfunction can manifest as a variety of problems and may include impairments in language or communication, impairments in motor function, and neuropsychiatric problems. Since the development of the central nervous system is involved, the noted difficulties may be apparent in infancy or childhood.

Examples include autism spectrum disorder (ASD), ADHD, and learning disorders. ASD comprises a group of neurodevelopment disorders that may be characterized by repetitive and characteristic patterns of behavior. In addition, individuals with ASD may exhibit difficulties with communication and social interactions. The symptoms are typically present from early childhood. According to the National Institute of Neurological Disorders and Stroke, ASD affects 1 in 65 children.

ASD is subdivided further into Asperger's syndrome, pervasive developmental disorder not otherwise specified, and autism.

Asperger's Syndrome

Asperger's syndrome is named for Hans Asperger, an Austrian pediatrician, who first described the condition in 1944. Asperger described a clinical series of four boys who showed uncoordinated or clumsy movements, dominant conversation tendencies, lack of empathy, and inability to form close friendships. He also detailed positive attributes of these individuals, including the increased ability to focus on details, strong independent work attitudes, original way of thinking, and the recognition of patterns that most others do not see.

Schizophrenia

Schizophrenia, as described by the National Institute of Mental Health, is a chronic and severe mental disorder that affects how a person thinks, feels, and behaves. People with schizophrenia are often described as losing touch with reality. Schizophrenia is not a condition of having a split personality or multiple personalities. This misconception likely originated from the 1960 movie. Schizophrenia is a chronic condition requiring lifelong treatment.

Individuals with schizophrenia often exhibit symptoms that are classified as either positive or negative symptoms. Positive symptoms are typically those that are psychotic in nature and appear to reflect an excess or distortion of normal functions. The diagnosis of schizophrenia, according to DSM-V, requires at least 1-month duration of two or more positive symptoms. Positive symptoms may include hallucinations, delusions, and thought and movement disorders.

Hallucinations are when one sees or hears something that does not exist. Hallucinations can be in any of the senses, but hearing voices (auditory hallucinations) are the most common type. *Delusions* refer to false beliefs that are not based in reality. Thought disorders may exhibit as communication that is disjointed, commonly referred to as "world salad." Movement disorders are agitated body movements.

Negative symptoms typically affect emotions and behaviors. Negative symptoms include the following: flat affect, difficulty staying on task, and anhedonia (reduced feelings of pleasure). Negative symptoms often persist in the lives of people with schizophrenia during periods of low or absent positive symptoms.

Schizophrenia is not a curable disease, but it is treatable. Antipsychotic medications can help treat the positive symptoms associated with the disorder. Psychosocial treatments can address the negative symptoms associated with this disorder. In addition, family education, cognitive behavioral therapy, and self-help groups can also help manage the condition.

Bipolar Disorder

Bipolar disorder includes alternating episodes of mania (excessive activity, energy, and excitement) with episodes of depression. Bipolar disorder affects approximately 5.7 million adult Americans, or about 2.6% of the U.S. population age 18 and older every year.[1] The median age of onset for bipolar disorder is 25 years, although the illness can start in early childhood or as late as the 40s and 50s.[2] The disorder is found equally in males and females.

The disorder is characterized by dramatic shifts in mood and energy levels that affect a person's ability to carry out daily tasks. The shifts in mood and energy levels are more severe than the normal ups and downs that everyone experiences. Manic periods may be characterized by periods of high energy, which may have individuals making significant plans, demonstrating pressured speech, and engaging in risky behaviors. The behaviors may include financial risks/high spending or sexual risks.

The depressive symptoms may consist of individuals showing low energy with depressive symptoms. They may feel sad, sleep a lot more, feel overwhelmed, and increase their eating. The increased eating may consist of increasing carbohydrate intake.

The disorder is treated with medications, including lithium and Abilify®. In addition, counseling can help individuals with symptoms and management. According to the surgeon general's report on mental health, consumers with bipolar disorder face up to 10 years of coping with symptoms before getting an accurate diagnosis, with only 1 in 4 receiving an accurate diagnosis in less than 3 years.

Depressive Disorders

Depressive disorders affect how individuals feel emotionally, such as the level of sadness and happiness, and can disrupt their ability to function. Major depression is one of the most common mental disorders in the United States. Depression is the result of a chemical imbalance, which is believed to be a low level of serotonin. Serotonin is a neurotransmitter in the central nervous system. Researchers have found lower levels of serotonin in the brain stem and cerebrospinal fluid of suicidal individuals.

Suicide is a potentially preventable public health problem. The National Institute of Mental Health lists suicide as the 10th leading cause of death in the United States and estimates there are nearly 40,000 suicides per year. Males are 4 times more likely to take their lives than females. Suicide has an incredible toll on families and is believed to be preventable as there are usually warning signs that a person is contemplating suicide. These are outlined below in Table 27.1.

Depression does respond to treatment. The American College of Physicians (ACP) performed an extensive systematic review of randomized controlled trials that evaluated treatments for depression from 1990 through late 2015.[3] Interventions that were evaluated included psychotherapies, omega-3 fatty acids, S-adenosyl-l-methionine, St. John's wort, exercise, and second-generation antidepressants. Following the extensive review, the ACP recommended that clinicians select between either cognitive behavioral therapy or second-generation antidepressants to treat patients with major depressive disorder.

Anxiety Disorders

Anxiety is an emotion characterized by fear. It may involve the anticipation of future misfortune. It is usually accompanied by excessive worrying. People with an anxiety disorder may develop avoidance behaviors. Examples of various anxiety disorders include generalized anxiety disorder, panic disorder, and phobias.

TABLE 27.1   WARNING SIGNS FOR SUICIDE

Always talking or thinking about death

Clinical depression—deep sadness, loss of interest, trouble sleeping and eating—that gets worse

Having a "death wish"

Losing interest in things one used to care about

Making comments about being hopeless, helpless, or worthless

Putting affairs in order, tying up loose ends, changing a will

Saying things like "It would be better if I wasn't here" or "I want out"

Sudden, unexpected switch from being very sad to being very calm or appearing to be happy

Talking about suicide or killing oneself

Source: National Institute of Mental Health.[4]

Panic disorder, as noted by the National Institute of Mental Health, affects about 6 million American adults and is twice as common in women as men. Panic attacks typically begin in late adolescence or early adulthood. Genetics are felt to play a role in the development of panic attacks. One will experience a feeling of being out of control during a panic attack. Such attacks are described as extremely fearful episodes. One will then begin to develop a worry about the potential for future attacks. This fear may translate into an avoidance of places where panic attacks have occurred in the past.

Physical symptoms are the hallmark of an attack. Individuals will describe a pounding or racing heart, difficulty breathing, sweating, chest or stomach pains, and a feeling of weakness. Repeated panic attacks can lead to a disabling condition of avoidance and even a withdrawal from public places. Some will become housebound due to their fears.

This condition is treatable. Mainstays of treatments are available including psychotherapy and medications. Psychotherapy will focus on cognitive behavior therapy. This technique will look to teach the person different ways of thinking, behaving, and reacting to situations that help him or her feel less anxious and fearful. Doctors also may prescribe medications to help treat panic disorder. The most commonly prescribed medications for panic disorder are anti-anxiety medications and antidepressants.

Trauma and Stressor-Related Disorders

Trauma and stressor-related disorders are adjustment disorders in which a person has trouble coping during or after a stressful life event. Examples include PTSD and acute stress disorder.

PTSD is a serious condition that can develop after a person has experienced or witnessed a traumatic or terrifying event in which serious physical harm may have occurred or had the potential to occur. PTSD is a lasting consequence of traumatic ordeals that cause intense fear, helplessness, or horror. PTSD can initiate from a traumatic event involving sexual or physical assault, the unexpected death of a loved one, an accident, war, or a natural disaster.

Symptoms of PTSD include reliving, avoiding, and increased arousal. Reliving is the repeated re-experiencing of the traumatic ordeal. It is usually accompanied by recurrent thoughts of the ordeal and may involve flashbacks, hallucinations, and nightmares. Avoiding occurs when a patient with PTSD avoids certain scenarios, people, or places that remind them of the trauma. This can lead to isolation. Increased arousal includes excessive emotions that then lead to problems such as relationship difficulties, sleep disturbances, and irritability.

Treatments that are typically utilized include medications and psychotherapies. The serotonin medications used to treat depression are also used to treat PTSD. Psychotherapies include cognitive behavioral therapies and exposure therapies. Exposure therapies involve having the individual relive the traumatic experience in a very controlled manner. Exposure therapy helps the person confront the fear and gradually become more comfortable with situations that are frightening and cause anxiety. This has been very successful in treating PTSD. In addition, family and group therapy has also been shown to be effective in treating PTSD.

NEED TO KNOW

Research trials are ongoing for a number of mental health disorders. The trials may be evaluating a new medication or counseling intervention. To search for a clinical trial near you, you can visit ClinicalTrials.gov. This is a searchable registry and results database of federally and privately supported clinical trials. The website will give you information about the purpose of the trial, locations, and contact information.

References

1. Kessler, R. C., Chiu, W. T., Demler, O., & Walters, E. E. (2005). Prevalence, severity, and comorbidity of twelve-month DSM-IV disorders in the National Comorbidity Survey Replication (NCS-R). *Archives of General Psychiatry, 62*(6), 617–627.

2. Kessler, R. C., Berglund, P. A., Demler, O., Jin, R., & Walters, E. E. (2005). Lifetime prevalence and age-of-onset distributions of DSM-IV disorders in the National Comorbidity Survey Replication (NCS-R). *Archives of General Psychiatry, 62*(6), 593–602.

3. Qaseem, A., Barry, M. J., Kansagara, D., & Clinical Guidelines Committee of the American College of Physicians. (2016). Pharmacologic treatment of adult patients with major depressive disorder: A clinical practice guideline from the American College of Physicians. *Annals of Internal Medicine, 164*(5), 350–359. doi:10.7326/M15-2570

4. https://www.nimh.nih.gov/health/topics/suicide-prevention/suicide-prevention-studies/warning-signs-of-suicide.shtml

Resources

American Psychiatric Association—Webpage for a professional organization of psychiatrists dedicated to promoting mental illness awareness and treatment: https://www.psychiatry.org/; http://aspennj.org

Austim Speaks—Web site that covers all aspects of autism and its impacts, this link reviews Asperger Syndrome: https://www.autismspeaks.org/what-autism/asperger-syndrome

National Institutes of Mental Health—Link to the site devoted to mental health topics, specifically schizophrenia: https://www.nimh.nih.gov/health/topics/schizophrenia/index.shtml

28

Marijuana

Objective

▸ Review of marijuana and its effects on individuals and society

Recreational Drug Use

Recreational drug use occurs when a drug is used with the primary intention of altering the central nervous system to gain emotional pleasure. The drug may be legal or illegal. Most legal drugs are also controlled substances.

Marijuana

The plant *Cannabis sativa* is the source of marijuana. The active substances in the plant can be found in the leaves, flowers, and stems. The plant contains the mind-altering chemicals known as cannabinoids. Two active cannabinoids are delta-9-tetrahydrocannabinol (THC) and cannabidiol (CBD).

History

Recently, a number of states have legalized the use of marijuana for both medical and recreational purposes. It is interesting to know that marijuana has been legal in the United States for the most of the country's history. Marijuana was recognized for its medicinal uses in the

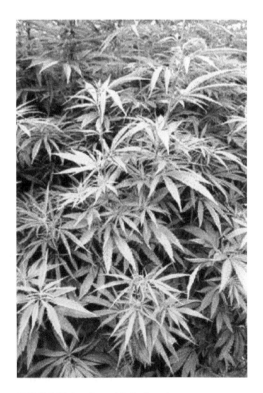

FIGURE 28.1 Cannabis Sativa plant.

mid-1800s. In fact, cannabis was included in the *United States Pharmacopoeia* for nearly 100 years.

Most historians feel that the Mexican Revolution was a factor in viewing marijuana in a negative light. The press described the negative concerns over Mexican immigrants and linked the use of marijuana to them. Congress realized that marijuana held the potential for revenue in the form of taxes. The Marihuana Tax Act of 1937, Pub. 238, 75th Congress, 50 Stat. 551 was a U.S. act that placed a tax on the sale of cannabis. The act was introduced to Congress on April 14, 1937. The act is now commonly known by the modern spelling as the 1937 Marijuana Tax Act.

Harry J. Anslinger, commissioner of the Federal Bureau of Narcotics, responded to political pressure to ban marijuana at a nationwide level. The Marihuana Tax Act of 1937 created an expensive excise tax and included penalty provisions and elaborate rules of enforcement to which marijuana, cannabis, or hemp handlers were subject. Mandatory sentencing and increased punishment were enacted when Congress passed the Boggs Act of 1952 and the Narcotics Control Act of 1956.

In *Leary v. United States* (1969), the Supreme Court held the Marihuana Tax Act to be unconstitutional since it violated the Fifth Amendment to the Constitution, which protects against self-incrimination. In response, Congress passed the Controlled Substances Act as Title II of the Comprehensive Drug Abuse Prevention and Control Act of 1970, which repealed the Marihuana Tax Act.

The Controlled Substances Act defined marijuana as a Schedule 1 substance. Schedule 1 substances as defined by the DEA and the U.S. Department of Justice meet three criteria. First, they are drugs or other substances that have a high potential for abuse. Second, the drug or other substance has no currently accepted medical use in treatment in the United States. Third, there is a lack of accepted safety for use of the drug or other substance under medical supervision. The federal government regards marijuana as an illegal substance.

Mechanisms of Action

THC acts on specific brain cell receptors. THC is very similar to naturally produced compounds in the body. These compounds play a role in normal brain development and function. Marijuana—and specifically THC—activates different areas of the brain that contain these receptors. Activation of these receptors can cause a variety of actions in the body; each action is dependent on the specific region of the brain that is activated. The specific areas of the brain and their functions are outlined in Table 28.1.

The Cerebral cortex is the area of the brain responsible for memory, thinking, and perception. THC can affect this area, leading to alterations in perception and affecting memory. Some individuals have reported that smoking marijuana can lead to the

TABLE 28.1   SPECIFIC BRAIN SITES AFFECTED BY MARIJUANA

Brain area	Function
Cerebral cortex	Plays a role in memory, thinking, perceptual awareness and consciousness
Hypothalamus	Governs metabolic processes such as appetite
Brain stem	Controls arousal, vomiting reflex, blood pressure, heart rate, and pain sensation
Hippocampus	Involved in memory storage and recall
Cerebellum	Responsible for coordination and muscle control
Amygdala	Plays a role in emotions

"munchies," which is due to the interaction of THC on the hypothalamus, the area of the brain responsible for appetite.

The brain stem is the area of the brain responsible for arousal, blood pressure, heart rate, and nausea/vomiting centers. THC may affect the brain stem by causing an increase in heart rate and inhibiting nausea/vomiting. It is thought that information from the stomach is sent to the nucleus of the solitary tract in the caudal hindbrain.[1] The hippocampus is the area of the brain involved in memory storage and recall. Marijuana can affect both memory storage and recall, at times invoking vivid flashbacks.

The cerebellum is the area of the brain responsible for coordination and muscle control. THC may impart coordination problems and difficulties with muscle control. Lastly, there are receptors in the amygdala. This center of the brain plays a role in emotions. The effects of marijuana may impact certain emotions. Cannabis has been shown to affect users' ability to recognize, process, and empathize with human emotions like happiness, sadness, and anger.[2]

Cognitive Effects

Marijuana also affects brain development. When individuals begin using marijuana as teenagers, the drug may reduce thinking, memory, and learning functions and affect how the brain builds connections between the areas necessary for these functions. One study showed that people who started smoking marijuana heavily in their teens and had an ongoing cannabis use disorder lost an average of 8 IQ points between ages 13 and 38. The lost mental abilities did not fully return in those who quit marijuana as adults. Those who started smoking marijuana as adults did not show notable IQ declines.[3]

MS is a neurological disease that may cause painful muscles spasms. Research has shown that the spasms may be reduced with marijuana use. However, MS is also associated with cognitive (thinking) difficulties. A well-controlled study determined that patients with MS who smoke cannabis are more cognitively impaired than nonusers with MS.[4]

Positive Effects

The National Institutes of Health has supported cannabis research to determine its potential positive effects on certain conditions and diseases. Since marijuana was illegal in the United States for a recent extended period, most medical claims were anecdotal. Recently, more about the potential medical effects of marijuana are being evaluated.

There is growing interest in the marijuana chemical CBD to treat certain conditions such as childhood epilepsy, a disorder that causes a child to seize. Therefore, scientists have been specially breeding marijuana plants and making CBD in oil form for treatment purposes. In addition, CBD is a cannabinoid that does not affect the mind or adversely affect behavior. According to the National Institutes of Health, CBD may be useful in reducing pain and inflammation, controlling epileptic seizures, and possibly even treating mental illness and addictions.

One recent animal study has shown that marijuana extracts may help kill certain cancer cells and reduce the size of others. Evidence from one cell culture study suggests that purified extracts from whole-plant marijuana can slow the growth of cancer cells from one of the most serious types of brain tumors. Research in mice showed that treatment with purified extracts of THC and CBD, when used with radiation, increased the cancer-killing effects of the radiation.[5] Research has not shown this to be true in humans at this time.

Glaucoma is a condition in which there is an abnormal buildup of intraocular (within the eye) pressure (IOP); if left untreated, this condition can lead to blindness. Research has found that smoking marijuana will lower the IOP. However, according to the American Academy of Ophthalmology, the IOP is only lowered for a short time, about 3 or 4 hours. Since the IOP needs to be lowered at all times, marijuana use would not provide the necessary coverage to treat this disease.

Currently, there are two cannabinoids (dronabinol and nabilone) or drugs approved by the FDA for the prevention or treatment of chemotherapy-related nausea and vomiting.

Negative Effects

Just as all medications have positive effects, they also have side effects or potential negative effects. We do know that marijuana can be addictive. Research suggests that about 1 in 11 users become addicted to marijuana and will seek it out on a daily or more frequent basis.[6,7]

Users also report less academic and career success. For example, marijuana use is linked to a higher likelihood of dropping out of school.[8] In addition, marijuana use has also been shown to lead to more job absences, accidents, and injuries.[9]

Marijuana smokers can develop a lung infection from a mold called aspergillosis, which is found on marijuana leaves. The mold may be inhaled when the marijuana leaves are smoked and inhaled. Some infections caused by mold are known as opportunistic infections, which refers to the fact that they will infect susceptible individuals. Typically, susceptible individuals have a weakened immune system. Immune systems are weakened in organ transplant patients, patients with AIDS, or patients recently receiving chemotherapy. In addition, medications used to treat inflammatory arthritis (rheumatoid or psoriatic) may also weaken the immune system. Aspergillus can cause an infection in the lungs (pneumonia) and even death. The American Thoracic Society does not recommend marijuana smoking in individuals with a compromised immune system.

Potpourri

As previously noted, more of the effects of marijuana use will be studied in the future. In January 2017 the National Academy of Sciences produced a paper detailing what we currently do know regarding the use of marijuana. The findings are summarized in Table 28.2. The drug will continue to provoke debates regarding both the positive and negative effects associated with its use.

TABLE 28.2   SUMMARY OF CURRENT RESEARCH REGARDING MARIJUANA USE

MS-related spasms and chemotherapy-induced nausea and vomiting are responsive to oral cannabinoids.

Use increases risk of being in a motor vehicle accident.

No increased risk of lung, head, and neck cancers.

Evidence suggests that cannabis smoking may trigger a heart attack.

Associated with more frequent bronchitis episodes, unclear if use increases other respiratory diseases.

Use is associated with an increased risk of developing schizophrenia.

Moderate evidence that use leads to increased tobacco, alcohol, and other illicit drug use.

Learning, memory, and attention are impaired directly after use.

Source: National Academy of Sciences, January 12, 2017.[11]

NEED TO KNOW

Legalization of marijuana is approved by a number of states for both medical and recreational usage. The benefits to the individualized states are obvious in regard to taxation benefits. The federal government also sees financial benefits in indirect ways.

  A recent study examined all prescriptions filled by Medicare Part D enrollees from 2010 to 2013 in 17 states and Washington, D.C., where marijuana is legalized. In these states, prescription drug use fell by 0.5%, with an estimated savings of $165 million in 2013 alone.[10] If the numbers are extrapolated, it is estimated that $470 million may be saved by Medicare Part D if marijuana use is approved by all 50 states.

References

1. Anthony, J., Warner, L. A., & Kessler, R. C. (1994). Comparative epidemiology of dependence on tobacco, alcohol, controlled substances, and inhalants: Basic findings from the National Comorbidity Survey. *Experimental and Clinical Psychopharmacology, 2,* 244–268.
2. Bradford, A. C., & Bradford, W. D. (2016). Medical marijuana laws reduce prescription medication use in Medicare part D. *Health Affairs, 35*(7), 1230–1236.
3. Cambridge, UK: Cambridge University Press.
4. Hall, W. D., & Pacula, R. L. (2003). *Cannabis use and dependence: Public health and public policy.*
5. Horn, C. C. (2008). Why is the neurobiology of nausea and vomiting so important? *Appetite, 50*(2–3), 430–434. doi:10.1016/j.appet.2007.09.015
6. McCaffrey, D. F., Pacula, R. L., Han, B., & Ellickson, P. (2010). Marijuana use and high school dropout: The influence of unobservables. *Health Economics, 19*(11), 1281–1299.
7. Meier, M. H., Caspi, A., Ambler, A. et al. (2012). Persistent cannabis users show neuropsychological decline from childhood to midlife. *Proceedings of the National Academy of Sciences, 109,* E2657–E2664.
8. National Academies of Sciences, Engineering, and Medicine. 2017. *The health effects of cannabis and cannabinoids: Current state of evidence and recommendations for research.* Washington, DC: The National Academies Press.
9. Pavisian, B., MacIntosh, B. J., Szilagyi, G., Staines, R. W., O'Connor, P., & Feinstein, A. (2014). Effects of cannabis on cognition in patients with MS: A psychometric and MRI study. *Neurology, 82*(21), 1879–1887. doi:10.1212/WNL.0000000000000446
10. Scott, K. A., Dalgleish, A. G., & Liu, W. M. (2014). The combination of cannabidiol and Δ9-tetrahydrocannabinol enhances the anticancer effects of radiation in an orthotopic murine glioma model. *Molecular Cancer Therapeutics, 13*(12), 2955–2967.
11. Troup, L. J., Bastidas, S., Nguyen, M. T., Andrzejewski, J. A., Bowers, M., & Nomi, J. S. (2016) An event-related potential study on the effects of cannabis on emotion processing. *PLoS ONE 11*(2), e0149764. Retrieved from https://doi.org/10.1371/journal.pone.0149764
12. Zwerling, C., Ryan, J., & Orav, E. (1990). The efficacy of preemployment drug screening for marijuana and cocaine in predicting employment outcome. *Journal of the American Medical Association, 264*(20), 2639–2643.

Resources

MedlinePlus—Webpage that updates medical uses for marijuana: https://medlineplus.gov/ency/patientinstructions/000899.htm

National Cancer Institute—Webpage that updates the latest possible uses of marijuana for cancer treatments: https://www.cancer.gov/about-cancer/treatment/cam/patient/cannabis-pdq

Figure Credit

Fig. 28.1: Copyright © Michael W (CC BY-SA 3.0) at https://commons.wikimedia.org/wiki/File:Cannabis_sativa.jpg.

29

Sexually Transmitted Diseases

Objectives

- ▶ Basic understanding of curable and treatable conditions
- ▶ Review of the most common sexually transmitted diseases and their symptoms, morbidity, and treatment

Conditions

The term *curable* applies to a disease or sickness that can be treated with either a drug or medicine and the problem will be brought to an end. *Treatable* is the medical term that indicates a disease or sickness is capable of being improved with a medicine or treatment. Treatable does not imply curable.

Latex Condoms

Latex condoms are applied to cover the penis and prevent the spread of semen (which contains sperm) from entering the female reproductive tract. The CDC reports that when latex condoms are used every time and put on early enough, they reduce chances of pregnancy over a 1-year period to 3%, compared with 85% without their use. Likewise, condoms cut the risk of human immunodeficiency virus (HIV) infection by about 80%, to less than a 1% chance of infection per year.

The condom acts as a barrier to prevent blood, semen, or vaginal fluids from passing from one person to the other during intercourse. Some diseases that are transmitted sexually are present in the semen, blood, or vaginal fluids and can pass from an infected individual, causing the partner to become infected. Condoms that are made of latex (rubber) or polyurethane for individuals allergic to latex have been shown to do the best job in terms of reducing the passage of HIV and hepatitis. The CDC warns that the package of the condom should state that the condoms are to prevent disease. This statement means the condom has passed a quality-control process. Other condoms that do not have his statement may be more of a novelty and may not meet basic standards of control to ensure adequate quality.

FDA inspectors perform a test on sample condoms they take from warehouses. The condoms are filled with water and checked for leaks. An average of 996 of 1,000 condoms must pass this test to meet quality-control standards. It should be noted that 4 out of 1,000 may not provide complete barrier protection.

Gonorrhea

Gonorrhea is an STD that is caused by the bacteria *Neisseria gonorrhoeae*. Gonorrhea is both treatable and curable. The risks of acquiring gonorrhea from an infected partner as estimated by CDC is 20% in males and 50% in females. The infection can cause a number of symptoms, but it is important to remember that up to 33% of women and 10% of men can have gonorrhea and exhibit no symptoms.

Symptoms associated with gonorrhea infection can affect multiple sites in the body. The rectum may be involved, especially in cases of anal sex involving penile–rectum penetration. Rectal infection may manifest with discharge from the rectum, bleeding, and anal itching. The eyes may also be involved. Gonorrhea can lead to photophobia (sensitivity to light), pain, and eye drainage. The joints of the body may also become infected, a condition that is not only very painful but also a medical emergency. Joint infection, also known as *septic arthritis*, requires immediate antibiotics and possible drainage of the infected joints.

In males, symptoms from gonorrhea infection may only be present 10% of the time. If symptoms are present, dysuria (pain when urinating) will be very common. Penile discharge may also be present; the color of the discharge can range from white to yellow to green. Less commonly, the testicles may be swollen or tender.

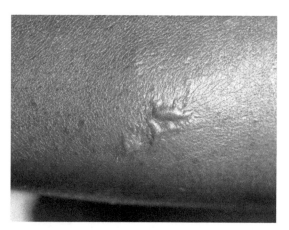

FIGURE 29.1   Gonococcal skin lesion.

Gonorrhea symptoms in females are present only about a third of the time, so most women will not have symptoms. The concern is that if left untreated, more serious complications will arise. These symptoms include dysuria, vaginal discharge, and vaginal bleeding outside of normal menses.

The diagnosis of gonorrhea can be done either by swabbing the endocervical region in women or urethral region in men. Alternatively, a blood test can also be performed. If the diagnosis is confirmed, then it is important to contact previous sex partners from the past 2 months for testing and possible treatment. Treatment is with antibiotics. The recommended antibiotics are ceftriaxone given as a single intramuscular injection or azithromycin given by mouth by a single dose.

If gonorrhea is left untreated in the female, pelvic inflammatory disease (PID) can occur. The gonorrhea infection can lead to collections of infected fluid (abscesses) to develop in the fallopian tubes. These are the tubes that connect the ovaries to the uterus. The ovaries release eggs for fertilization, which travel in the tubes and if fertilized will implant in the uterus. The infections can cause scar tissue, abscesses, and damage to the reproductive organs.

Complications may include infertility, chronic pain, and ectopic pregnancy. PID and repeated infections can increase the risk of infertility. The infections have a cumulative effect on infertility. PID is also associated with chronic lower abdominal or pelvic pain. PID may also be associated with dyspareunia (pain during intercourse). In addition, *ectopic pregnancy* refers to the fertilized egg not implanting in the uterus but in the fallopian tube. The failure to implant in the uterus may be due to a blockage of the fallopian tube. Ectopic pregnancies can be life-threatening emergencies that may require emergency.

Doctors diagnose PID based on signs and symptoms of the patient. They may also perform a pelvic examination. Diagnostic testing will also include an analysis of vaginal discharge and cervical cultures. Tests on urine will be done to rule out a urinary tract infection. Treatment for PID includes a course of antibiotics for both the patient and his or her partner and a period of abstinence to prevent reinfection.

Chlamydia

Chlamydia is an infection caused by the bacteria *Chlamydia trachomatis*. Chlamydia is both treatable and curable. It causes an infection of the cervix (cervicitis) in women. Men may get infections of the urethra (urethritis) or rectum (proctitis). The CDC notes that chlamydia is the most frequently reported bacterial sexually transmitted infection in the United States. In 2014, 1,441,789 cases of chlamydia were reported to CDC, but an estimated 2.86 million infections occur annually. Chlamydia is most common among young people. Almost two thirds of new chlamydia infections occur among youth aged 15–24 years. The CDC also estimates that 1 in 20 sexually active young women aged 14–24 years have chlamydia.

Chlamydia infections commonly involve the cervix, urethra, and eye. The infection is diagnosed via vaginal swab in women and urine specimen for men. The urine specimen is also an alternative method for testing in women. The treatment for infection is the same as for gonorrhea. The two bacteria are commonly found together. Doxycycline is used for bacterial resistant cases and is taken twice a day for 10 days.

HPV

While chlamydia is the most common bacterial infection, HPV is the most common sexually transmitted infection. It is caused by a virus. HPV is treatable but not curable. It is also potentially preventable. The virus will characteristically cause warts in the genital area. The genital warts usually appear as a small bump or group of bumps. They can range in size from small to large and can be flat to raised, or cauliflower in shape.

Diagnosis is typically made by a health care provider by visual examination of the warts. The warts can be treated. If the genital warts are left untreated, sometimes they will resolve on their own; they may stay the same or grow both in size and number. They are treated with a variety of options. Creams such as podofilox and imiquimod can be prescribed by a health care provider. They are intermittently applied to warts for a period of up to 4 weeks. The warts can be frozen off with liquid nitrogen, or be surgically resected. Electrocautery (application of an electric current) can also remove the warts. Lastly, they can be removed with use of a laser.

While the warts may be unsightly and embarrassing, it is important to remember that the types of HPV that can cause genital warts are not responsible for causing cancers. The high-risk types HPV 16 and 18 are responsible for approximately 70% of cervical cancers.[1] The low-risk nononcogenic HPV types 6 and 11, cause anogenital warts and recurrent respiratory papillomatosis.[2]

The major concern with HPV is that it can lead to cancers. Cervical cancer is the most common cancer, but it can also cause cancers of the vulva, vagina, penis, or anus. It is for this reason that it is recommended sexually active females be evaluated by health care providers on an annual basis. The doctor may take swab cells of the cervix to evaluate for the presence of HPV. If HPV—specifically, the subtypes associated with cancer—is found, then regular surveillance of the cervix and an annual PAP test may be done. The surface of the cervix may also be viewed using a special magnifying device, known as the colposcope, to perform a colposcopy, which looks closely for abnormal changes in the surface of the cervix, vagina, and vulva. The cancers often take years to develop.

The CDC reports among women diagnosed with an HPV cancer, cervical cancer is the most common, with about 11,000 women diagnosed annually in the United States; subsequently, about 4,400 women die every year from cervical cancer in our country. For men in the United States diagnosed with an HPV cancer, oropharyngeal cancer is the most common. Around 7,200 U.S. men each year are diagnosed with oropharyngeal cancer caused by HPV infection.

HPV infection may be preventable. HPV vaccines are available and are now routinely recommended for 11- and 12-year-old girls and boys. Vaccination is also recommended for females ages 13 through 26 years and males ages 13 through 21 years who were not vaccinated when they were younger. The CDC also recommends vaccination for both men who have sex with men and men aged 22 through 26 years who were not vaccinated when they were younger. The quadrivalent vaccine is directed against HPV 6, 11, 16, and 18; the bivalent vaccine is directed against HPV 16 and 18. The HPV vaccines are given in three shots over 6 months; as with any vaccination, it is important to get all three doses, as this will increase the chances of an effective response.

Research has evaluated the effectiveness of the HPV vaccines, finding vaccine efficacy against lesions related to the specific HPV types in the vaccine being 96% for cervical cancer, 100% for both vulvar and vaginal cancers, and 99% for genital warts. Vaccine efficacy against any lesion (regardless of HPV type) for cervical cancers was 30%.[3]

Genital Herpes

Genital herpes has historically been caused by the HSV-2 virus. Genital herpes is treatable but not curable. The CDC estimates that in the United States, about 1 out of every 6 people aged 14 to 49 years have genital herpes. It is also estimated that, annually, 776,000 people in the United States get new herpes infections. Nationwide, 15.5 % of persons aged 14 to 49 years have HSV-2 infection, and 80% don't know they have it. There are medicines that can treat, prevent, or shorten outbreaks, but no medicines to cure herpes.

Infections are transmitted through contact with lesions, mucosal surfaces, genital secretions, or oral secretions. HSV-1 and HSV-2 can also be shed from skin that looks normal. Generally, a person can only get an HSV-2 infection during sexual contact with someone who has a genital HSV-2 infection. Transmission most commonly occurs from an infected partner who may or may not have visible lesions or sores and commonly may not know he or she is infected.

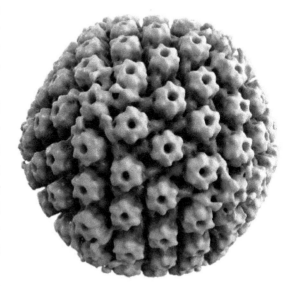

Genital herpes may be characterized by fluid-filled blisters on the genitals. Condoms do not provide reliable protection, as the virus is spread when it touches another person's skin. You can contract the virus even if there are no active blisters on the genitals. One study found that in 70% of patients, transmission appeared to result from sexual contact during periods of asymptomatic viral shedding.[4] Both early and late lesions can occur with herpes.

Treatment for genital herpes is done during symptomatic eruptions. The eruptions are more likely to occur during times of stress. On average, there are

FIGURE 29.2   3D reconstruction of herpes simplex virus 1 (HSV-1).

typically four to six flares per year. The flares are treated with antiviral medications. Valcyclovir or acyclovir are typically used to shorten the length of the flare.

HIV

HIV is a sexually transmitted virus that is treatable but not curable. HIV was first reported in the 1980s. The virus attacks white blood cells, specifically the T cells. These are the cells that the body uses to fight infections and provide surveillance against potential cancers. The diagnosis of HIV is done via a blood test. The test will look for specific antibodies that the body uses to fight the virus. It may take the body anywhere from 6 weeks to 1 year to develop the antibodies, thus producing a positive test result. Follow-up tests may be needed, depending on the initial time of exposure.

Early testing is crucial, as it permits early identification and early treatment. Treatments consist of a cocktail of medications that are known as combination antiretroviral therapy (ART). These medications will attack the human immunodeficiency virus at multiple stages of its life cycle. The medications of today are life-saving and life sustaining. Today a 20-year-old HIV-positive adult on ART in the United States or Canada is expected to live into his or her early 70s, a life expectancy approaching that of the general population.[5]

Syphilis

Syphilis is an STD that is caused by the bacteria *Treponema pallidum*. Syphilis is treatable and curable. The CDC estimates that in 2014 that there were 63,450 reported new cases of syphilis. The syphilis rate is on the increase among the male homosexual population, as this group accounted for 83% of all new cases reported. Syphilis can be transmitted from person to person via direct contact with a syphilitic sore. The sore is known as a chancre. Chancres occur mainly on the external genitals, vagina, anus, or rectum. They can also occur on the lips and in the mouth. Their location is dependent on the type of sex being performed.

Transmission of syphilis occurs during vaginal, anal, or oral sex. Pregnant women with the disease can transmit it to their unborn child. Syphilis can be cured with the right antibiotics from your health care provider. However, treatment will not undo any damage that the infection has already done. Previous or past infection does not prevent future infection. Long-term complications can occur if not treated correctly.

Symptoms in adults are divided into stages: primary, secondary, or latent. The *primary stage* may be characterized by a single or multiple sores or chancres. The sore is located where syphilis entered the body. The sore is usually firm, round, and painless. The sore lasts 3 to 6 weeks and heals regardless of whether the person receives treatment. Even though the sore goes away, individuals must still receive treatment so the infection does not move to the secondary stage.

During the *secondary stage*, patients may have skin rashes and/or sores in the mouth, vagina, or anus (also called mucous membrane lesions). This stage usually starts with a rash on one or more areas of the body. The rash can show up when the primary sore is healing or several weeks after the sore has healed. The rash can look like rough, red, or reddish-brown spots on the palms of the hands and/or the bottoms of the feet. The rash is not itchy. The symptoms from this stage will go away whether or not you receive treatment. Without treatment, the infection will progress to the latent stage of syphilis.

The *latent stage of syphilis* may begin after individuals have had syphilis for years and without active signs or symptoms. Most people with untreated syphilis do not develop latent stage syphilis. Symptoms of the latent stage of syphilis include difficulty coordinating your muscle movements, paralysis (not able to move certain parts of your body), numbness, blindness, and dementia (mental disorder with an inability to remember). There is also the potential for damage to one's internal organs and even death.

NEED TO KNOW

Less Risky Sex Versus Safe Sex

Marketing campaigns advocate using condoms for safe sex. "Safe" implies it is without risks. It's important to know, however, that condoms cannot completely protect you and your partner from some STDs. According to the National Institutes of Health, condoms are impervious to the smallest viruses. Condoms, however, can break or slip off 1% to 2% of the time. The use of petroleum-based products (such as Vaseline) for lubrication can cause breakdown of the latex condom. Additionally, surveys show most people don't use condoms properly or consistently, and roughly 12 million Americans each year contract an STD.

Individual studies have shown that the transmission rates for various STDs differ greatly. None of the transmission rates drop to 0% with the use of condoms. One study examined the transmission rate for women in acquiring gonorrhea and chlamydia from infected males and showed the use of condoms will produce a 62% reduced risk of acquiring gonorrhea and a 26% reduction in the risk of acquiring chlamydial infection.[6] Another study followed adolescent African American females and combined incidence of gonorrhea, chlamydial infection, or trichomoniasis and found the girls who reported using condoms developed at least one STD at a rate of 17.8% compared with a rate of 30% in the girls who did not report using condoms consistently.[7] The effectiveness of condoms in protecting against HPV infection and HPV-related conditions such as genital warts and cervical cancer has also been evaluated. A meta-analysis of 20 studies found no evidence that condoms were effective against genital HPV infection.[8] Another study followed 444 female college students looking at the incidence of genital HPV infection. The study found that consistently using condoms with a new partner was not associated with significant protection against HPV.[9] HIV transmission rates with condom use have also been studied. It is thought that condom use will reduce the risk of transmission of HIV by 80%, with a range of 35% to 94%.[10] The difference in protections rates may be related to the specific type of STD tested. Some are viral in origin, and others are bacterial. For HPV, intimate contact prior to sexual intercourse may allow for spread of the virus to the hands and then to the genitals. Similar transmission of the bacterial infections of gonorrhea and chlamydia can occur after intimate touching and before sexual intercourse.

It is important to remember that if you develop symptoms previously discussed in this chapter and consistently use condoms, you are still at risk for an STD. Regular—and as needed—evaluation by your physician to address concerns and to avoid long-term complications of STDs is recommended.

References

1. Crosby, R. A., DiClemente, R. J., Wingood, G. M., Lang, D., & Harrington, K. F. (2003). Value of consistent condom use: A study of sexually transmitted disease prevention among African American adolescent females. *American Journal of Public Health, 93,* 901–902.

2. de Sanjose, S., Quint, W. G., & Alemany, L. et al. (2010). Human papillomavirus genotype attribution in invasive cervical cancer: A retrospective cross-sectional worldwide study, *Lancet Oncology, 11,* 1048–1056.

3. FUTURE I/II Study Group, Dillner, J., Kjaer, S. K., Wheeler, C. M. et al. (2010). Four year efficacy of prophylactic human papillomavirus quadrivalent vaccine against low grade cervical, vulvar, and vaginal intraepithelial neoplasia and anogenital warts: Randomised controlled trial. *BMJ, 341,* c3493. doi:10.1136/bmj.c3493

4. Lacey, C. J. N., Lowndes, C.M., & Shah, K. V. (2006). Burden and management of non-cancerous HPV-related conditions: HPV-6/11 disease. *Vaccine, 24*(S3), 35–41.

5. Manhart, L. E., & Koutsky, L. A. (2002). Do condoms prevent genital HPV infection, external genital warts, or cervical neoplasia? A meta-analysis. *Sexually Transmitted Diseases, 29,* 725–735.

6. Mertz, G. J. et al. (1992). Risk factors for the sexual transmission of genital herpes. *Annals of Internal Medicine, 116*(3), 197–202.

7. Samji, H., Cescon, A., Hogg, R. S., Modur, S. P., Althoff, K. N., Buchacz, K. et al. (2013). Closing the gap: Increases in life expectancy among treated HIV-positive individuals in the United States and Canada. *PLoS ONE, 8*(12), e81355. Retrieved from https://doi.org/10.1371/journal.pone.0081355

8. Sanchez, J., Campos, P. E., Courtois, B., Gutierrez, L., Carrillo, C., Alarcon, J. et al. (2003). Prevention of sexually transmitted diseases (STDs) in female sex workers: Prospective evaluation of condom promotion and strengthened STD services. *Sexually Transmitted Diseases, 30,* 273–279.

9. Weller, S., & Davis, K. (2004). *Condom effectiveness in reducing heterosexual HIV transmission. Issue*

10. Winer, R. L., Lee, S.-K., Hughes, J. P., Adam, D. E., Kiviat, N. B., & Koutsky, L. A. (2003). Genital human papillomavirus infection: Incidence and risk factors in a cohort of female university students. *American Journal of Epidemiology, 157,* 218–226.

Figure Credits

Fig. 29.1: Source: https://commons.wikimedia.org/wiki/File:Gonococcal_lesion_on_the_skin_PHIL_2038_lores.jpg.

Fig. 29.2: Copyright © Thomas Splettostoesser (CC BY-SA 4.0) at https://commons.wikimedia.org/wiki/File:HSV-1-EM.png.

30

Medicare and Medical Assistance

Objectives

▸ Basic understanding of Medicare
▸ Basic understanding of Medicaid

Terms

Insurance plans, terms, and conditions can be confusing and not well understood. It is important to understand the different terminologies of the insurance industry. *Premium* is the term given to the monthly fee that is paid to a health plan/insurance company for health coverage. A lower premium is preferred to a higher one. *Deductible* is the term used to describe the amount you will need to pay out of pocket before your health insurance plan begins to pay. Therefore, it is in the best interest of the consumer to have a low deductible; for example, if your deductible is $1,000, you will need to spend $1,000 before your insurance plan will begin to cover medical costs. Obviously, a deductible of $1,000 is preferable to a deductible of $3,000.

History

The idea of a federally funded insurance program had been discussed for a few decades. President Lyndon Johnson made it a priority during his term as president. Johnson's goal was to begin a federally funded insurance program for the elderly in America. He envisioned the program being able to provide low-cost medical and hospital care for the elderly. According to the LBJ Presidential Library, half of the country's population over age 65 had no medical insurance, and a third of the aged lived in poverty, unable to afford proper medical care.

Johnson's idea of a national insurance program for the elderly met resistance from the AMA. The majority of physicians would not support such a plan. Johnson sought the support of the AMA in a different program to rotate physicians in and out of Vietnam to serve the civilian population. When the AMA agreed to this plan, the LBJ Presidential Library describes the following:

Johnson ordered an impromptu press conference, in which he praised the AMA for its commitment to the Vietnam War. When asked inevitably about whether the AMA would support Medicare, Johnson declared, "These men are going to get doctors to go to Vietnam where they may be killed. Medicare is the law of the land. Of course, they'll support the law of the land." He then turned to the AMA president, "You tell him." Put firmly on the spot, he replied, "Of course, we will. We are law abiding citizens, and we have every intention of obeying the new law." Within a matter of weeks, the AMA would formally endorse Medicare, with 95 percent of doctors not resisting it but following suit.[1]

Johnson traveled to the Harry S. Truman Library and Museum in Independence, Missouri, where Truman, and his wife, Bess, watched Johnson sign Medicare into law on July 30, 1965. Johnson credited Truman with starting the idea during his presidency decades before and awarded the first two Medicare cards to Truman and his wife.

Over the years, Congress has made changes to Medicare. The changes have expanded the coverage, allowing more people to become eligible. In 1972 Medicare was expanded to cover the disabled, people with end-stage renal disease requiring dialysis or kidney transplant, and people 65 or older who select Medicare coverage.

The Children's Health Insurance Program (CHIP) was created in 1997. The intent of the program was to cover uninsured children. The initial program, according to the Centers for Medicare & Medicaid Services, provided health insurance and preventive care to nearly 11 million uninsured children in America. The children were from families of the "working poor," uninsured families that had earned too much to be eligible for Medicaid. Currently, all 50 states and the District of Columbia have CHIP plans. It is a federal program that is run on the individual state level.

The Medicare Prescription Drug, Improvement, and Modernization Act of 2003 (MMA) made the biggest changes to the Medicare program in 38 years. It was signed into law under President George W. Bush. The MMA created and acknowledged private health plans. These plans are known as Medicare Advantage Plans and are referred to as Medicare Part C. The MMA also expanded Medicare to include an optional prescription drug benefit. This was signed into law under President George W. Bush and went into effect in 2006. The Medicare prescription plan is known as Medicare Part D.

The Patient Protection and Affordable Care Act, commonly called the Affordable Care Act (ACA) and commonly referred to as "Obamacare," was signed into law by President Barack Obama in 2010. It represented the most significant changes to Medicare and Medicaid since their inception in 1965. The ACA created the Health Insurance Marketplace, a single place where consumers can apply for and enroll in private health

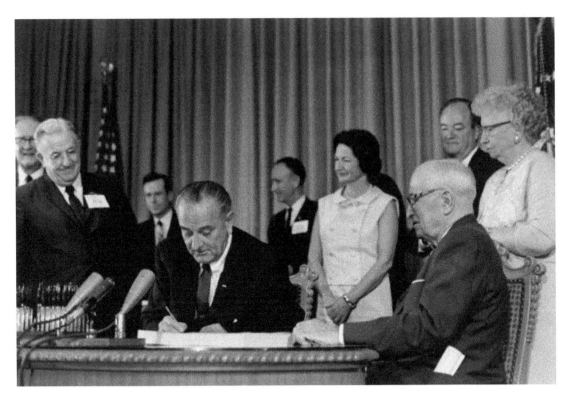

FIGURE 30.1   President Lyndon Johnson signs the Medicare Bill at the Harry S. Truman Presidential Library.

insurance plans. It also expanded coverage by raising the minimum income levels for individuals and families and eliminating insurers' ability to discriminate or deny insurance based on preexisting conditions. It also allowed children to be covered on a parent's insurance plan until the age of 26 years. Additional provisions of the act focused on tax penalties for the uninsured.

Organization

When enacted, Medicare was the responsibility of the Social Security Administration, and Medicaid was the responsibility of the Social and Rehabilitative Service Administration. Both were part of the U.S. Department of Health, Education, and Welfare. The department was reorganized in 1980; the U.S. Department of Health and Human Services (HHS) was created, and Medicare and Medicaid became known as the Centers for Medicare & Medicaid Services (CMS), and they report to the secretary of HHS.

Medicare is a health insurance program for people age 65 and older. It may also provide coverage and services for individuals under age 65 with certain disabilities, patients with end-stage disease, or patients with amyotrophic lateral sclerosis, also known as Lou Gehrig's disease. It consists of four parts: Medicare Part A, B, C, and D.

Medicare Part A

Medicare Part A is hospital insurance. Part A helps cover inpatient care provided in hospitals as well as skilled nursing facilities. It also helps cover hospice care and some home health care. Beneficiaries must meet certain conditions to get these benefits. There is typically no monthly premium required for Medicare Part A, provided that either you or your spouse paid Medicare taxes while working.

You usually don't pay a monthly premium for Medicare Part A (hospital insurance) coverage if you or your spouse paid Medicare taxes while working. The original idea of Medicare was to pay in while working. Part A is largely funded by revenue from a 2.9% payroll tax levied on employers and workers (each pay 1.45%). Individuals in business for themselves will be responsible for the entire 2.9%. Beginning in 2013 the rate of Part A tax on earned income exceeding $200,000 for individuals ($250,000 for married couples filing jointly) rose to 3.8%, in order to pay part of the cost of the subsidies mandated by the ACA. The taxes will need to have been paid for a period of 10 years. If the taxes have not been paid, one may purchase Medicare Part A at monthly premium of up to $411 each month.

Associated Medicare Part A costs include deductibles and coinsurance. The deductibles and coinsurance amounts are listed in Table 30.1. Medicare pays hospitals and health care systems using a prospective payment system. This system provides the health care institution with a set amount of money for each episode of care provided to a patient. The amount of money is a fixed amount and not based on the actual amount of care provided to the patient. The hospital can make money if it spends fewer resources (orders fewer tests, shorter length of stay) and conversely lose money if it spends more

TABLE 30.1   MEDICARE PART A DEDUCTIBLES AND COINSURANCE

For Part A hospital inpatient deductible and coinsurance, you pay:	$1,288 deductible for each benefit period
Days 1–60	$0 coinsurance for each benefit period
Days 61–90	$322 coinsurance per day of each benefit period
Days 91–151	$644 coinsurance per each "lifetime reserve day" after day 90 for each benefit period (up to 60 days of your lifetime reserve days)
Beyond 60 lifetime reserve days	all costs

Source: cms.gov.[3]

resources on the patient. The money is based on the diagnosis the patient received when admitted to the hospital, which is known as the diagnosis related group (DRG).

To keep the system in check and to prevent substandard care and premature discharges, Medicare penalizes hospitals for readmissions. If a patient is readmitted to a hospital within 30 days of a hospital admission, Medicare will then recover any payments made to the hospital for the patient's initial stay as well as a penalty of between *4 to 18 times* the initial payment amount. The total penalties for above-average readmissions in 2013 are $280 million, for 7,000 excess readmissions, or $40,000 for each readmission above the U.S. average rate.[2]

Medicare Part B

Part B is medical insurance. This part will help cover physician's services and outpatient care. It also covers some other medical services, such as the services of physical and occupational therapists, and some home health care. It also covers the cost of supplies (durable medical equipment) when they are medically necessary. Part B premiums vary by income. The lowest an individual will pay is $104.90 each month. The actual amounts are detailed in Table 30.2.

After your deductible is met, you typically pay 20% of the Medicare-approved amount for most doctor services. These physician services include either inpatient or outpatient visits with the doctor. They also include outpatient therapy and durable medical equipment.

TABLE 30.2   MEDICARE PART B PREMIUMS

File Individual Tax Return	File Joint Tax Return	File Married and Separate Tax	You Pay Each Month (2017)
$85,000 or less	$170,000 or less	$85,000 or less	$134
Above $85,000 up to $107,000	Above $170,000 up to $214,000	Not applicable	$187.50
Above $107,000 up to $160,000	Above $214,000 up to $320,000	Not applicable	$267.90
Above $160,000 up to $214,000	Above $320,000 up to $428,000	Above $85,000 and up to $129,000	$348.30
Above $214,000	Above $428,000	Above $129,000	$428.60

Source: Medicare.gov[4]

Medicare Part C

Medicare Part C is also known as the Medicare advantage plan. With the passage of the Balanced Budget Act of 1997, Medicare beneficiaries were formally given the option to receive their Original Medicare benefits through capitated health insurance Part C plans, instead of through the Original fee for service Medicare payment system. The premium varies by plan. Medicare beneficiaries who choose this option do not have the traditional Part A and Part B. Their Medicare C plan covers both Part A and Part B costs and services. There are a number of factors to consider when choosing a Medicare advantage plan. Some plans may offer gym or health club memberships, prescription plans, or lower premiums. It is important to remember that the Medicare advantage plan may have a smaller network, have higher deductibles, and lack a nationwide network.

There are some publications that rank the plans and other sites that can help determine which plan may be the best for an individual to choose. The choice should be based on the current and anticipated medical needs.

Medicare Part D

Prescription drug coverage is provided under *Medicare Part D*. This part was added due to the increasing costs of prescription medications. Medicare Part D is available to everyone with Medicare. This coverage is to help lower prescription drug costs and to protect against higher costs in the future. People will pay a monthly premium for this coverage. The monthly premiums are based on income and are noted in Table 30.3. While Medicare Part D has helped lower prescription drug costs, concerns over a gap in coverage known as the *donut hole* has proven frustrating for participants. The current system of coverage may require Medicare Part D or Medicare advantage plan enrollees to assume 100% of the cost of the drug until their yearly deductible is met, this can be considered the deductible phase. The initial coverage phase follows, the enrollee

TABLE 30.3   MEDICARE PART D PREMIUMS

File Individual Tax Return	File Joint Tax Return	You Pay (In 2017)
$85,000 or less	$170,000 or less	Your plan premium
Above $85,000 up to $107,000	Above $170,000 up to $214,000	$13.30 + your plan premium
Above $107,000 up to $160,000	Above $214,000 up to $320,000	$34.20 + your plan premium
Above $160,000 up to $214,000	Above $320,000 up to $428,000	$55.20 + your plan premium
Above $214,000	Above $428,000	$76.20 + your plan premium

Source: Medicare.gov.[5]

TABLE 30.4   MEDICARE PART D COVERAGES

Phase	Threshold	Costs
Deductible	Until deductible is met	100% of medications
Coverage	Until $3,750	Plan's costs
Coverage gap (donut hole)	Until $5,000	35% brand name and 44% generics
Catastrophic Coverage	No limits	5% of medications

will pay their share according to their plan, until $3,750 has been spent. The coverage gap or donut hole phase then begins, during this time the patient will need to pay 35% of the cost of brand name drugs and 44% of the cost of generic drugs. This phase will end when the patient pays a total of $5,000 of medication costs. The catastrophic coverage phase begins and the patient is then only responsible for 5% of the cost of their medications. Table 30.4 summarizes the coverage issues with Medicare Part D.

President Trump's 2018 budget will end the donut hole in 2019, with Medicare Part D enrollees paying a flat 25% of the cost of medications. [Table 30.4]

Medicare Supplemental Insurance

Medigap plans are private health insurance plans sold to supplement Medicare. Medigap insurance provides coverage for many of the copays and some of the coinsurance related to Medicare plan. The name is derived from the notion that it exists to cover the difference, or gap, between the expenses reimbursed to providers by Medicare Parts A and B. Medigap plans are available to participants in Medicare Parts A and B. Participants in Medicare Part C or the Medicare Advantage Plans are not eligible for the Medigap plan. The Medicare website can be a very valuable resource in determining which plan is offered in your area. It also lists which plans will cover hospice care, foreign travel, blood, skilled nursing services, and out-of-pocket limits. The choice of obtaining a Medigap plan as well as the specific Medigap plan should be based on one's current and anticipated medical needs.

Medicaid

When Medicaid was enacted into law in 1965, it provided medical insurance to people getting cash assistance or the very poor. The program has been expanded over the years. Today a much larger group is covered: low-income families, pregnant women, individuals with disabilities, and people who require long-term care. CHIP covers children. According to the Medicaid website, 74,550,529 individuals were enrolled in

Medicaid and CHIP in the 50 states and Washington DC reporting May 2017 data. Medicaid covers roughly 23% of the American population. Medicaid is a hybrid federal–state program. The federal government sets minimum guidelines for Medicaid eligibility, but states can choose to expand coverage beyond the minimum threshold. The individual states can adjust the programs to best serve the people in their state. For this reason, there is a wide variation in the services offered from state to state.

Issues of concern exist with the Medicaid plan, including the escalating costs to provide coverage to nearly 75 million Americans. Some physicians and other health care providers do not accept patients with Medicaid insurance. They choose not to participate in their state's program secondary to the low payment or reimbursement rates that the state through its Medicaid program pays to providers for services rendered to patients. This varies from state to state. There is also a feeling of greater patient noncompliance issues that further frustrate health care providers. These issues will need to be resolved, as this program has expanded and continues to do such.

NEED TO KNOW

Durable medical equipment is covered under Medicare Part B. One example is a transcutaneous electrical nerve stimulation unit (TENS). TENS units can be very helpful in helping reduce muscular or nerve-based pain. Medicare has traditionally reimbursed medical vendors up to $600 for such units. If your physician writes a prescription for a unit, and the prescription is taken to a medical supply or equipment business, they may bill Medicare or your insurance company $800 for such a unit, leaving you with a copay of $200 or more. Very similar units can be purchased online for about $29 to $49. The cheaper units are effective. They can also save the patient or consumer a significant amount of money.

References

1. Updegrove, Mark K. *Indomitable Will: LBJ in the presidency.* Crown Pub, 2012.
2. Summary of costs and benefits.(2012). *Federal Register.* Retrieved from https://www.federalregister.gov.
3. https://www.cms.gov/Newsroom/MediaReleaseDatabase/Press-releases/2016-Press-releases-items/2016-11-10-2.html
4. https://www.medicare.gov/your-medicare-costs/part-b-costs/part-b-costs.html
5. https://www.medicare.gov/part-d/costs/premiums/drug-plan-premiums.html

Resources

Centers for Medicare & Medicaid Services (CMS)—Main homepage for the Medicare and Medicaid services, starting point for having your questions answered with numerous links exploring all aspects of the programs: https://www.cms.gov/

LBJ Presidential Library—Website to learn further perspectives on the history of Medicare and Medicaid and President Johnson's roles in the programs: http://www.lbjlibrary.org/

Figure Credit

Fig. 30.1: Source: https://commons.wikimedia.org/wiki/File:LyndonJohnsonSigningMedicareBill.gif.

Insurance Issues

Objective

> ▸ Basic understanding of the medical insurance world and its impact on consumers

I N ORDER TO best understand the world of medical insurance, it is imperative that you understand the terms associated with insurance plans. It is not only vital to know what the various terms mean, but also to understand how they will affect both you and your family.

Premium

Premium is the term given to the monthly fee that is paid to a health plan/insurance company for health coverage. The lower the premium, the less money you will need to pay for coverage. The premiums charged by insurance companies or by health plans continue to increase yearly. The yearly increases exceed the annual inflation rate. Certain companies may charge higher premiums to people who make more money and lower premiums to people who make less money. This model moves toward a socialistic approach for medicine. Sometimes, it may be difficult to know what your monthly premium is, especially if you have direct deposit service for your wages. Your company's human resources department should be able to answer questions in regard to your monthly premium.

Deductible

Deductible is the term used to describe the amount you will need to pay out of your pocket before your health insurance plan begins to pay. Therefore, it is in your best interest to have low deductibles; for example, if your deductible is $1,500, you will need to spend $1,500 before your insurance plan will begin to cover medical costs. Obviously, the lower the deductible, the less out-of-pocket costs are absorbed by the consumer.

Coinsurance

Coinsurance refers to your share of the costs of a covered health care service. Coinsurance can be calculated as a percentage (for example, 20%) of the allowed amount for the service. You are able to pay your coinsurance amount only after you've met your annual deductible. For example, if the health insurance plan's allowed amount for an office visit is $100 and you've met your deductible, your 20% coinsurance payment would be $20. The health insurance plan pays the rest.

Allowed Amount

Allowed amount is the maximum amount on which payment is based for covered health care services. This term may appear on your health care summary or on your bill. Allowed amount may also be called "eligible expense," "payment allowance," or "negotiated rate." If your health care provider charges more than the allowed amount, you may be responsible for paying the difference.

Consolidated Omnibus Budget Reconciliation Act

The Consolidated Omnibus Budget Reconciliation Act (COBRA) is a federal law that allows for employees to temporarily keep health coverage after their employment ends. The coverage may be extended for themselves or their family (dependents) for a period of up to 18 months. COBRA coverage allows you to keep the same insurance plan you had with your company when you were working. You, however, will be responsible for paying the entire premium plus an additional administrative fee. While employed, your employer may have paid for some or all of your premium during your employment, so it is very likely your costs to maintain insurance will increase.

Copayment

Copayment is a fixed amount you pay for a covered health care service, usually after you receive the service. The copayment amount can vary by your particular insurance plan as well as the service provided. Your insurance card may list the copayment amounts on your insurance card. The amounts owed will vary according to the service provided and may include office visit to a primary care provider, office visit to a specialist, ER visit, preventive services, and mental health services.

Flexible Spending Account

A flexible spending account (FSA) is an arrangement you set up through your employer to pay for many of your out-of-pocket medical expenses. These expenses include insurance copayments as well as deductibles and qualified prescription drugs and medical devices. The advantage of such a plan is that the money put into an FSA account is tax free. The employer's plan will set a limit on the amount you can put into an FSA each year. One disadvantage to an FSA is that there is no carryover of FSA funds year to year. Some plans may have a 2½-month grace period after the end of the FSA year. Such a plan can be helpful for individuals with fairly fixed and predictable medical costs over a 12-month period. The savings occur when the money that is placed in the FSA is not taxed. It can save consumers the total amount of money at the level of their income tax rate. For example, if they have $400 in fixed medical costs per month, they will put $4,800 into an FSA. If they are also in the 18% income tax bracket, they will save 18% of $4,800, or $864 in 1 year.

Health Savings Accounts

Health savings accounts (HSAs) were created in 2003 for individuals with high-deductible health plans to save money for medical expenses. The money placed into an HSA is similar to an FSA in that it is tax free. Individuals can receive tax-preferred treatment of money saved for medical expenses. Unlike FSAs, the plan is individually owned. The plan is are also portable if you change jobs. One can deposit money into an HSA, where it earns interest tax free. Funds are not taxed when they are used for qualified medical expenses. The federal government sets annual limits to amount for HSAs. In 2016 the limits were $3,350 for individuals and $6,750 for a family. The deadline for contributions to an HSA are the same as an IRA, (April 15 of the following year). Anyone can make contributions to your HSA, including yourself, family members, or your employer. The contributions may be a one-time contribution, deposits throughout the year, or automatic deductions from paychecks. In addition, individuals can use an IRA to contribute to their HSA; it can only be done once in their lifetime and must not exceed the annual contribution limit.

There are different insurance products and plans. Occasionally, consumers may be locked into a specific plan that is the only one offered by their employer. Different options regarding the care level, premiums, and deductibles may exist. Other times consumers may need to decide between completely different plans.

Health Maintenance Organization

A health maintenance organization (HMO) is a type of health insurance plan that usually limits coverage to care from doctors who have a contract with the HMO. It generally won't cover out-of-network care except in an emergency. An HMO may require you to live or work in its service area to be eligible for coverage. HMOs often provide integrated care and focus on prevention and wellness. HMO plans tend to have very low premiums and lower deductibles. It does require the insured to obtain a primary care physician (PCP). The plan will usually require individuals to get a referral from their PCP to see a specialist. For this reason, the PCP may be referred to as a "gatekeeper." The plan may have a very limited network and may not cover out-of-network services.

Preferred Provider Organization

A preferred provider organization (PPO) is a health plan that contracts with medical providers such as hospitals and doctors to create a network of participating providers. You pay less if you use providers that belong to the plan's network. You can use doctors, hospitals, and providers outside of the network for an additional cost. You are typically not required to obtain a PCP. This type of plan is typically more expensive than other plans. It does allow the consumer more freedom for choices of providers and services.

Point of Service Plan

A point of service plan (POS) is a plan in which you pay less if you use doctors, hospitals, and other health care providers that belong to the plan's network. POS plans also require you to get a referral from your primary care doctor in order to see a specialist. POS plans typically will allow for out-of-network coverage. The POS plan is considered to be a cross between an HMO and PPO plan. Costs for a POS plan tend to run higher than an HMO plan.

Insurance Issues

Most patients feel that they have great insurance plans, until the time comes to use them. When they need to use the plan, they may be in for a reality check. Insurance rules can be frustrating to patients and providers alike. There have been numerous reports of patients being denied care and necessary services because of their specific health care plan allowances. From a provider's prospective, the insurance industry can be equally frustrating.

One frustration the provider may experience is the credentialing process. It may take weeks to months before plans will credential a provider into their network. During this time of awaiting credentialing, the provider can decline seeing patients in that particular insurance plan or see the patients without financial reimbursement. Seeing patients without the services being billable, certainly does not incentivize the insurance company to credential the provider in a timely fashion.

Another frustration of providers is the denial of services. It can be frustrating for providers to sign a contract to care for patients in that they are trying to provide care and may get denial of services from the insurance plan. Another frustration providers may experience is the insurance plan may not provide certain benefits for the patient. The benefits may be a procedure to help a patient's pain or a medication that may not be covered by the patient's insurance plan.

The world of medical insurance continues to change and evolve. Premium costs continue to climb. Deductibles also show annual increases. Change is one constant in life, and insurance plans will continue to change.

NEED TO KNOW

"Peer-to-peer review" is the term given to the insurance process of an appeal. When the insurance company denies a particular service, the treating physician can request a peer-to-peer review. This is when the treating physician will discuss the details of the case on behalf of the patient in an attempt to get the service covered by the insurance company. Sometimes the peer-to-peer review can be successful, but other times the denial is upheld. Consumers can ask their physician to request a peer-to-peer review in an attempt to get a particular service, medication, or imaging study approved.

Electronic Medical Records

Objectives

- ▸ Basic understanding of electronic medical records
- ▸ Discussion of how electronic medical records have and will impact patient care

Electronic Records

Electronic records may refer to either the electronic medical record or the electronic health record. These records are different and may contain different content. The electronic medical record (EMR) contains the standard medical and clinical data gathered in one provider's office. The electronic health record (EHR) is more comprehensive. The EHR may contain and share information from all providers involved in a patient's care. According to HealthIT.gov, EHR data can be created, managed, and consulted by authorized providers and staff from across more than one health care organization.

According to the U.S. Department of Health & Human Services, the Health Information Technology for Economic and Clinical Health (HITECH) Act enacted as part of the American Recovery and Reinvestment Act of 2009 was signed into law on February 17, 2009. The intention of the law is to promote the adoption and meaningful use of health information technology. The HITECH Act also addresses the privacy and security concerns associated with the electronic transmission of health information. It provides several provisions that strengthen the enforcement of The Health Insurance Portability and Accountability Act of 1996 (HIPAA). HIPPAA established national standards to ensure the security and privacy of health information and security guidelines for electronic protected health information (e-PHI) and its transmission and exchange.

Paper Medical Chart

Historically, patients' medical records were contained in their medical chart. The chart was a folder that contained medical information. This medical information included: the lab/test results, insurance information, radiology reports, operative notes and office notes. The sections were included in the patient's medical chart. The physician would write pertinent information into the chart from the patient's appointment. The information from the visit would include the patient's chief complaint (reason for visit), current symptoms, and physical examination findings. The office note would also contain the diagnosis and outline the plan of treatment.

The medical chart would typically be divided into sections and in chronological order. When the patient's chart exceeded a certain number of pages, a new volume would be created. Some patients may have multiple volumes. The charts required dedicated physical space in the office. They also needed to be readily accessible. The medical charts also required some degree of security or limited access and lastly, the medical information needed to remain confidential.

The electronic medical record is a virtual chart; it is not a physical chart or folder. The chart is accessible on computer and requires hard drive or computer memory for storage. All information in the EMR needs to be entered into the chart. The inputted information is not free from errors, although the information entered is legible. Initially, it was believed that the EMR is more secure. With backup capability, it was not thought to be vulnerable to fire, flood, or other physical damage/loss. However, data security and medical information specifically have become prime hacking targets. There have been a number of breaches concerning patient information, from hacking to loss of laptops containing private patient information. The main differences between the two charts are summarized in Table 32.1.

The CMS believes that EMRs can improve patient care in a number of areas. EMRs will reduce the incidence of medical error by improving the accuracy and clarity of medical records. EMRs make health information readily available, reduce duplication of tests, reduce delays in treatment, and allow patients to be more informed to make better decisions. The best way to inform patients is via the patient–physician interaction.

Reducing medical errors by improving the accuracy and clarity of medical records is also a focus of the EMR. The use of EMRs is expected to reduce errors in medical records. There is no doubt that handwritten records are subject to lots of human errors due to misspelling, illegibility, and differing terminologies. The use of EMRs may permit standardization of patient health records. One such area where there is no debate with accuracy is with handwritten prescriptions. The Institute for Safe Medication Practices produces a list of more than 300 medications that can be confused for one another. The list has medications that either are spelled alike or sound alike.

TABLE 32.1   DIFFERENCES BETWEEN TRADITIONAL CHART AND EMR

Traditional Chart	EMR
Paper chart	Virtual chart
Requires physical space	No physical space
Storage issues	Digital storage issues
Security concerns	Security concerns
Physical writing in chart (legibility issues)	Data entered as typed notes
Stored all office medical information	Stored all office medical information

The ones that are spelled alike are a concern with handwritten prescriptions. For example, one medication doxycycline, is an antibiotic used to treat Lyme disease and other infections. It is usually written for 100mg. Another medication that has been confused for doxycycline is doxepin; this medication is used to treat depression, anxiety, and sleep disorders. It is also written for 100mg dosage. The risk to patients is getting doxepin when they should be receiving doxycycline, their Lyme disease or other infection will not be adequately treated. If the patient erroneously receives doxycycline instead of doxepin their mental health concerns will not be adequately addressed.

The medications that sound alike may also present a problem. This occurs when prescriptions are called in over the phone from a physician's office to the pharmacy. The problem is often a result of the physician or office leaving a message at the pharmacy regarding the prescription, as the medication sound may be misinterpreted. This potential error is less likely to occur if the physician or health care provider speaks directly to the pharmacist. It is also important for consumers to check the literature they receive with their prescriptions to ensure the proper medication has been attained.

Pros

Paper records can be easily lost. Medical offices and hospitals have had fires, floods, and other natural occurrences that have destroyed the physical records of patients. The argument for digital records is they can be stored virtually forever. EMRs can also consolidate records in one place. It is not uncommon for older medical records to be archived and kept off-site, since physical storage in the office may be limited. In addition, EMRs can have built-in action plans to ensure certain medications or necessary testing is performed. This may include immunizations, laboratory testing, mammograms, and colonoscopies.

Cons

There is some concern that EMRs may threaten privacy. Depending on how they are arranged, records may list every diagnosis past and present on the patient's main screen. This may include a mental health diagnosis or other emotionally sensitive ones to the patient. The patient may not be comfortable seeing this on the screen during a visit for a completely unrelated reason, especially for a relatively minor medical issue.

EMRs can lead to loss of the "human touch" in health care. In the process of digitalization, the interpersonal aspect in health care may be lost. In handwritten hospital charts and office notes, doctors and other health care practitioners would chart or write their personal observations regarding their interactions with the patients in their own words. EMRs are arranged in a way to use prepopulated comments via using drop-down menus and clicking on boxes. Physicians can find the electronic chart difficult to interpret, as the note will contain significant amounts of computer-generated lists of medications and diagnosis.

EMRs are not efficient. Some EMR programs are not considered user-friendly. These programs may require multiple steps and the need to confirm each step to perform a relatively simple order in the chart. This is in direct contrast to being able to order almost any product in the world through an online shopping site with one click. A 2014 survey of the American College of Physicians member sample, however, found that family practice physicians spent 48 minutes more per day when using EMRs. Ninety percent reported that at least one data management function was slower after EMRs were adopted, and 64% reported that note writing took longer. Over a third (34%) reported that it took longer to find and review medical record data, and 32% reported that it was slower to read other clinicians' notes.[1] The results of this study are not compatible with one of the reported intentions of the EMRs.

Conversion

In an attempt to expedite conversion to EMR in hospitals, doctor's offices, and health care systems, the federal government offered financial incentives to help offset the costs of conversion. In order to receive the maximal incentive, providers needed to participate in 2011. The incentives turned into financial penalties in 2015 for Medicare and Medicaid providers who did not transition to EHRs. Highlights of the incentive program are noted in Table 32.2.

TABLE 32.2   EHR INCENTIVE PROGRAM HIGHLIGHTS

Maximum EHR incentives are $44,000 over 5 consecutive years.

EHR incentive payments decrease if starting after 2012.

Must begin by 2014 to receive EHR incentive payments; last incentive payment year is 2016.

Extra amount available for providers practicing in predominantly health professionals shortage areas.

Eligible hospitals including critical access hospitals (CAHs) can qualify for EHR incentive payments totaling some $2 million or more.

Meaningful Use

Meaningful use is a federal government (CMS) program that uses certified EHR technology to improve patient care and clinical outcomes. According to HealthIT.gov, meaningful use looks to improve quality, safety, and efficiency and reduce health disparities. It also works to engage patients/family and improve care coordination in population and public health. It is also thought that the meaningful use program and EHRs will maintain better privacy and security of patient health information. Ultimately, CMS hopes that the meaningful use compliance will result in better clinical outcomes, improved population health outcomes, increased transparency and efficiency, empowered individuals, and more robust research data on health systems.

The meaningful use program was launched in 2011 and introduced as a three-stage process. Stage 1 focused on data capture and sharing, tracking of key clinical conditions, initiating the reporting of clinical quality measures and public health information, and using the information to engage patients and their families in their care.

Stage 2 of meaningful use was instituted in 2014. It focused on an increase in health information exchange, increased requirements for e-prescribing, better incorporation of lab results, more controlled patient data, and the electronic transmission of patient summaries across multiple settings.

The current and third stage of meaningful use was started in 2016. It emphasizes improvement in quality, safety, and efficiency; patient access to self-management tools; and access to comprehensive patient data through patient-centered health information exchange. The stages of meaningful use are summarized in Table 32.3.

The meaningful use program emphasizes core measurements. They are to be assessed with each visit. The core measurements include a problem list of the patient, medications, allergies, vital signs, and smoking status of the patient. Critics argue that asking and then needing to document the status in a 70-year-old nonsmoker during each visit may take away time from addressing more immediate concerns.

The impacts of EMR and meaningful use have led to less of a face-to-face interaction with patients. The physician or health care provider may be focused with entering data into the EMR in order to comply with regulations. The associated costs to maintain an IT department may be significant, as well as paying for and implementing upgrades to the system. The landscape of medicine has been changing as more physicians and health care providers are employed by hospitals and health care systems and fewer are in a private practice model. The stresses and costs associated with EHRs may be a factor in this trend.

Another concern with the meaningful use program is its rigid criteria. In a letter addressed to CMS's Patrick Conway, the acting principle deputy administrator of the American Hospital Association (AHA) explains that the agency needs to leave behind its "all-or-nothing" approach to doling out incentive payments, noting that eligible hospitals and eligible providers may lose out on their entire incentive payments by failing to meet only one meaningful use requirement. The AHA wants meaningful use to be a more flexible program, allowing hospitals and providers who have met 70% of requirements to be categorized as meaningful users.

TABLE 32.3   MEANINGFUL USE STAGES

Stage 1 (2011–2012)

Data capture and sharing
Standardized format
Track key clinical conditions
Communication for care coordination processes
Initiating the reporting of clinical quality measures and public health information
Using information to engage patients and their families in their care

Stage 2 (2014)

More rigorous health information exchange
Increased requirements for e-prescribing and incorporating lab results
Electronic transmission of patient summaries across multiple settings
More patient controlled data

Stage 3 (2016)

Improving quality, safety, and efficiency, leading to improved health outcomes
Decision support for national high-priority condition
Patient access to self-management tools
Access to comprehensive patient data through patient-centered health information exchange

The U.S. Government Accountability Office (GAO), according to its website, is an independent, nonpartisan agency that works for Congress. Often called the congressional watchdog, the GAO investigates how the federal government spends taxpayer dollars. The GAO recently completed an evaluation of the Veterans Health Administration (VA) medical sites. The evaluation found the following: Pharmacists cannot electronically exchange prescriptions with non-VA providers and pharmacies. Therefore, veterans need to obtain paper prescriptions from external providers, have the providers fax the prescriptions from external providers, or have the providers fax the prescriptions to their local VA pharmacy to fill the prescriptions, which is time-consuming and inefficient. The VA is limited in its ability to interoperate with private providers. The GAO recommends the VA system assess the impact of interoperability. The physicians and health care providers for the federal insurance plans Medicare and Medicaid are expected to have and utilize electronic prescribing (e-prescribing) or face financial penalties, but if they treat a veteran in the VA system they will be unable to e-prescribe (which can lower their e-prescribing percentages) and potentially place them at risk of federal monetary penalties.

References

1. McDonald, C. J., Callaghan, F. M., Weissman, A., Goodwin, R. M., Mundkur, M., & Kuhn, T. (2014). Use of internist's free time by ambulatory care electronic medical record systems. *JAMA Internal Medicine, 174* (11), 1860–1863.

Resources

HealthIT.gov—Site that outlines the meaningful use program for providers: https://www.healthit.gov/providers-professionals/ehr-incentive-programs

Institute for Safe Medicine Practices—Website that has an astounding list of sound alike medications that may present consumers with potential problems: http://www.ismp.org/Tools/confused-drugnames.pdf

U.S. Department of Health & Human Services—Webpage that outlines the various aspects of HITECH act: https://www.hhs.gov/hipaa/for-professionals/special-topics/HITECH-act-enforcement-interim-final-rule/index.html

Government Accountability Office—Homepage of the government accountability office a watchdog group that analyzes spending for congress, they specifically issued the report on VA prescriptions: https://www.gao.gov/about/

33

Internet Searches

Objectives

- ▸ Basic understanding of MEDLINE
- ▸ Basic knowledge of research studies
- ▸ Understanding of good medical Internet sites

MEDLINE

MEDLINE is the U.S. National Library of Medicine (NLM) premier bibliographic database. According to the NLM, MEDLINE contains more than 22 million references to journal articles in life sciences, with a concentration on biomedicine. MEDLINE is the online counterpart to MEDLARS® (Medical Literature Analysis and Retrieval System) that originated in 1964. MEDLINE is part of the Entrez series of databases provided by the NLM National Center for Biotechnology Information. MEDLINE will typically cover articles from 1946 to present. Over the past decade, 2,000 to 4,000 completed references have been added each day.

Medical journals contain articles, commentaries, and reviews that look to further advance our understanding of medicine. The articles may serve to review a medical topic, thoroughly reviewing the current understanding of a disease. The article will describe the particular disease in terms of etiology, cause, diagnosis, and treatments. Other articles in medical journals may describe the results of a new or novel treatment focusing on the outcomes of such treatments. Commentaries will offer opinions on a particular topic. Many consumers may be surprised to know that opinions on treatment approaches do not always achieve a 100% consensus.

Historically, medical journals have been published and are similar to magazines in terms of size and quality of the binding and pages. Recently, journals are being accessed more and more electronically. Journals may reach or impact all physicians and have a national or international reputation. Some popular medical journals in this genre include *New England Journal of Medicine* (NEJM),

Journal of the American Medical Association (JAMA), and the *British Medical Journal (BMJ)*. Other medical journals that may be directed to a particular specialist include the journals *Spine* and *Chest*.

Research Studies

Research is of vital importance to our understanding of medicine. The research study may evaluate the effectiveness of a treatment, try to determine causality of a particular disease, or describe a potential new treatment approach. There are different types of research studies, and the types may fall under a hierarchy in terms of their importance. Not all research gets published. Certain scientific standards are typically met when a study is published in a journal. Many journals will require a peer review process. The editorial staff is made up of physicians, many of whom are leaders in their field of medicine. The journal may have the article *peer reviewed* by these physicians. This is the process that ensures a basic standard for published research.

There are different research studies that can be performed. Animal research, case report study, case control study, cohort study, randomized controlled trial, systematic review, and meta-analysis are the different types that will be reviewed. They are presented in order from lesser to a greater level of evidence (significance). It is important for consumers to have a basic understanding of the different studies as the marketing departments will highlight the fact that their products have been "scientifically shown" to work. Positive results in an animal research study or a case report study are much different than results published in a RTC or meta-analysis.

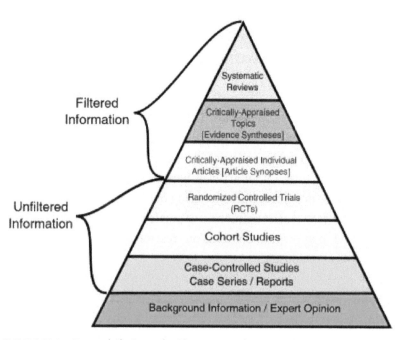

FIGURE 33.1   Research design and evidence pyramid.

Animal Research

Animals may be the initial testing focus of a novel device, medicine, or medical procedure. Testing on animals is done for the purpose of determining the effects of the potential treatment. For medicine testing, the emphasis will be on the effects of the medicine as well as its potential damage to the body (toxicology). Medicine testing will be done on animals and if without toxic effects will then proceed to Phase 1 testing on humans. Animal testing is also done to evaluate a medical device. The artificial heart, or left ventricular assist device, was implanted in the 1980s during its developmental stage in cows before testing commenced in humans. The device was approved by the FDA for clinical use in humans in 2008. The medical procedure of a bone marrow transplantation was done initially in animals before earning researchers Dr. Joseph E. Murray and Dr. E. Donnall Thomas the Nobel Prize in Physiology or Medicine in 1990. They were jointly awarded the prestigious award "for their discoveries concerning organ and cell transplantation in the treatment of human disease." According to the Health Resources and Services Administration (HSRA), this potentially lifesaving procedure is performed on an estimated 19,000 patients per year.[1]

Case Report Study

A *case report study* is a report that focuses on a single patient and his or her disease, treatment, and outcome. The placebo response associated with pain is 30%, so this factor should be kept in mind. Additionally, different individuals can respond quite differently to medicines. The differences include both the medication's efficacy (success rate) and its side effects. The case report study is valuable in the sense that if a new treatment is successful and the article allows others to know of the treatment, further testing and investigation may be done to confirm the initial claims.

Case Control Study

A *case control study* is a research study that essentially works backward. The study will begin looking at a particular outcome or disease that has occurred in a group of individuals and then looks for potential causes. It will compare a group of individuals who have the disease with a group of individuals who do not have the disease. The study will then work backward (retrospectively) to find if a certain exposure is associated with the disease. For example, it may take a group of patients with colon cancer and compare them to a group of patients without colon cancer and ask them both about their diet, specifically their intake of fats. The researchers may be able to note that the group with a higher intake of saturated fat was 4 times more likely to develop colon cancer than the group that had a lower intake of saturated fat in their diet.

Strengths of the case control study include low cost, short in study length, ability to evaluate multiple exposures at the same time, and good at initiating a potential association. Limitations of this type of study are bias, as the study relies on memory (those with the disease may be more prone to better recall risk factors); inadequate for studying rare diseases; and this type of study is only able to examine a single outcome.

Cohort Study

A *cohort study* follows a group over an extended period of time and analyzes risk factors or exposures to determine which in the group gets a certain disease. This type of study is usually done on a prospective basis. The landmark cohort study is the Framingham Heart Study. This study was started in 1948 by a group of researchers looking to identify risk factors for heart disease. The study is still ongoing and is sponsored by the National Heart, Lung, and Blood Institute and Boston University. The Framingham Heart Study has immensely improved our understanding of heart disease and risk factors. Thanks to the study, we now know the following: Cigarette smoking was found to increase the risk of heart disease (1960), high blood pressure was found to increase the risk of stroke (1970), high levels of HDL (good) cholesterol were found to reduce the risk of death (1988), progression from high blood pressure to heart failure was described (1996), and sleep apnea is tied to increased risk of stroke. This is an abbreviated list of the more than 33 significant findings that have been discovered.

Randomized Control Trial

A *randomized control trial* (RCT) is a study in which subjects are randomly chosen to receive one of several clinical interventions. The study may frequently be done without the subject knowing the particular intervention that they are receiving (blind RCT). The strength of such research is in the randomization process. Physicians may also refer to this study as the "gold standard", in that when done correctly is very convincing in terms of treatment efficacy (effectiveness). Examples of an RCT may be testing of a new medication for high blood pressure. The subjects are split into two groups: A and B.

Group A is assigned the experimental medicine to lower blood pressure. Group B is assigned a placebo tablet (control group). Both groups do not know whether they are given the medicine or placebo (blind RCT). Their blood pressure is monitored and recorded for 3 months. The results are analyzed for both groups. The researchers will determine if Group A had better control of their blood pressures with the experimental medicine compared to Group B, which received the placebo. The results can then be published, advancing the possible treatments for high blood pressure.

Systematic Review

A *systematic review* is a research paper that will summarize the results of previously published studies. The systematic review will typically summarize well designed health care studies (controlled trials). When the studies are reviewed together they collectively can provide a high level of evidence. The higher level of evidence can then provide better clarity to the efficacy of the medications or interventions allowing for better recommendations for physicians and health care providers.

Cochrane is associated with performing systematic reviews. Cochrane is a global independent network of researchers, professionals, patients, caregivers, and people interested in health. According to its website, it has 37,000 contributors from more than 130 countries. They work together to produce credible, accessible health information that is free from commercial sponsorship and other conflicts of interest. They produce Cochrane Reviews to achieve this goal, producing reviews on a variety of medically related topics. Their stated mission is to provide accessible, credible information to support informed decision making, which has never been more important or useful for improving global health.

Meta-analysis

A *meta-analysis* is similar to a systematic review in that it combines previously published studies and reviews the results. The main difference is that the meta-analysis will incorporate a statistical procedure that integrates the results of several independent studies considered to be "combinable."[2] The meta-analysis will then look to statistically derive a conclusion based on the analysis. The benefits of meta-analysis include a consolidated and quantitative review of a large, and often complex, sometimes apparently conflicting, body of literature.[3] Given the extensive amount of ongoing research and its availability to search and review online, this type of study is now feasible.

Searches

MEDLINE is the primary component of PubMed (http://pubmed.gov); a link to PubMed is found on the NLM homepage (http://www.nlm.nih.gov). The result of a MEDLINE/PubMed search is a list of citations (including authors, title, source, and often an abstract) to journal articles and an indication of free electronic full-text availability. Searching is free of charge and does not require registration. A growing number of MEDLINE citations contain links to the free full text of the article archived in PubMed Central™ or to other sites.

Consumers can search terms to determine if research studies may support claims they are hearing or reading about. To search, one needs to enter the key words of the search into PubMed. For example, if you want to know if green tea lowers the risk of cancer, you would enter "green tea," "cancer," and "reduction" into the search. The result will be a list of studies in chronologic order (newest first). If you wish to evaluate a study further, you would simply click on it. You will likely get an abstract (summary) of the study and a link to the entire study. For most consumer cases, reading of the abstract will likely be sufficient; and if not, there is usually a link to the article. Sometimes the link will be for free access to the article, but other times the link will require payment for viewing of the article. The articles are written in scientific language, but the main point of the article will be summarized in fairly easy-to-understand language in the conclusion (last) section of the abstract. The method(s) section of the abstract will define the type of study as well as the number of subjects involved. This will help put the results in their proper perspective or significance.

NEED TO KNOW

Most Americans are aware of the health benefits of eating oats. Studies have shown the consumption of oats will lower cholesterol. Labels for breakfast oats will draw attention to this fact with a picture of a heart or a statement noting this fact. Do Americans know how much eating oats will lower their cholesterol? What does the research show? The original study was titled "The Effect of Rolled Oats on Blood Lipids and Fecal Steroid Excretion in Man." Patricia A. Judd and A. Stewart Truswell were the authors, and it was published in 1981 in the *American Journal of Clinical Nutrition*. The abstract states the following: "Plasma total cholesterol concentrations were reduced in seven of 10 subjects, but over the whole group the mean reduction of 8% was not significant (0.05 less than p less than 0.01)."[4] A meta-analysis was completed in 1992 and published in *JAMA*. The findings of that study showed a reduction of 5.9mg/dL.[5] The research confirms that eating oats will likely reduce one's cholesterol, but not to a significant degree.

References

1. https://bloodcell.transplant.hrsa.gov/research/transplant_data/transplant_activity_report/index.html
2. Egger, M., Smith, G. D., & Phillips, A. N. (1997). Meta-analysis: Principles and procedures. *BMJ, 315*(7121), 1533–1537.
3. Haidich, A. B. (2010). Meta-analysis in medical research. *Hippokratia, 14*(Suppl. 1), 29–37.
4. Judd, P. A., & Truswell, A. S. (1981). The effect of rolled oats on blood lipids and fecal steroid excretion in man. *American Journal of Clinical Nutrition, 34*(10), 2061–2067.
5. Ripsin, C. M., Keenan, J. M., Jacobs, D. R., Jr. et al. (1992). Oat products and lipid lowering: A meta-analysis. *Journal of the American Medical Association, 267*(24), 3317–3325.

Resources

Cochrane—Homepage for Cochrane a group of researchers that examine the evidence and allows for informed decisions regarding medical treatments form their statistical reviews: http://www.cochrane.org/about-us

Framingham Heart Study—Website for the long running research study and efforts of Boston University and the National Heart, Lung and Blood Institute: https://www.framinghamheartstudy.org/

National Library of Medicine—Home of the National Library of Medicine, with links for PubMed, MedlinePlus, toxic information and clinical trials: https://www.nlm.nih.gov/

Figure Credit

34

Internet Claims

Objectives

- ▸ Brief review of the impact of the Internet on medicine
- ▸ Basic understanding of how to find good medical information
- ▸ Review of helpful medical Internet sites
- ▸ Better understanding of Internet claims

Innovation

Historically, doctors have embraced and created new technology to advance patient care. Technology has allowed physicians to repair a problematic heart valve without opening the chest, repair a torn ligament with the use of an arthroscope, or treat painful kidney stones with the use of soundwaves (lithotripsy). The Internet is technology that has affected many levels of medicine.[1] The Internet has nearly unlimited information. Traditionally, patients would be seen in a doctor's office and be given a diagnosis and information. The information was given either as verbal information or printed information in the forms of pamphlets or information sheets. The patient would accept the information given and follow the instructions.

Now anyone can search the Internet for medical information. Consumers can now visit many of the sites that inform and educate doctors. Popular search engines can find scholarly journals, slide presentations, or clinical guidelines. Consumers and patients can also visit chat rooms and blogs. The sites can be beneficial in some cases and problematic in others.

Another example of how the Internet has changed medicine is with the use of web portals. These are sites where patients can access their health records and lab results or communicate with their health care providers. This ability can be beneficial to patients if they are concerned about the results of a particular test or study, and the results may reassure them. It also has the potential to be problematic. For example, a patient has a complete blood count (CBC) done to evaluate for a potential underlying lung infection during an asthmatic flare. The CBC results are accessible on the patient web portal site. The results indicate an increase in the patient's white blood cell count (WBC). The patient then Google elevated WBCs. The search will list infections and cancers as potential causes. The patient then worries about leukemia, when the true cause was an elevated WBC count secondary to the patient taking a course of steroids for asthmatic exacerbation.

Physician Access

Physicians will also use the Internet to keep informed. They may receive their journal subscriptions online, reviewing articles in the journal to keep their knowledge base current. There are also online subscription services that are available for a fee. One such service is UpToDate. The health care provider can search a particular medicine, disease, or diagnosis on this site and will get information regarding the inquiry. The frequency, etiology, presenting symptoms, and treatments for the disease will be readily available.

E-mail exchanges between patients and providers are also a result of changes in ongoing communication. Consumers may be able to e-mail specialists around the world regarding symptoms and treatment options. There have been suggestions of e-medicine, in which the face-to-face communication is done online to evaluate, assess, diagnose, and treat conditions. Most physicians will still prefer the person-to-person interaction to practice medicine. Medicine is more of an art than a science.

Dr. Google

A great deal of patients will use the search engine Google to begin their search of symptoms to make a diagnosis of their medical problems. How accurate is such a practice? In terms of diagnostic accuracy, this question was answered by two Australian specialists.

In 2006 they tested the diagnostic accuracy of Google searches by entering symptoms and signs from 26 published case records. The search revealed the correct diagnosis in 15 cases and the incorrect diagnosis in the remaining 11 cases.[2] They found Internet searching was more effective for conditions with unique symptoms and signs. Complex diseases with nonspecific symptoms or common maladies with rare presentations were less likely to be diagnosed correctly.

What can you possibly learn from your health care provider that is not available on the Internet? Sir Francis Bacon is credited with the saying "knowledge is power." This is very true, but also know that knowledge is not wisdom. Physicians and other health care providers are in the best position to weigh information and advise patients, drawing on their understanding of available evidence as well as their training and experience.[1]

Patients who perform an online search of a disease will receive the search results. The results can sometimes be commercially influenced. The search will not differentiate from the most likely to the least likely possibilities. For example, say a consumer search "low back and leg pain." The resulting terms will yield various sites and links. The consumer may get locked into a less likely diagnosis of piriformis syndrome rather than the more likely lumbar disc causes. He or she may then search for treatments of the incorrect diagnosis causing further delay in the appropriate treatments or the potential for a worsening of his or her ongoing condition. The health care provider will then need to spend additional time convincing the person of the correct diagnosis and dispelling the incorrect one.

Domains

The domain name is part of the uniform resource locator (URL) used to access websites. The top level domain (TLD) name is located just to the right of the web address. Common TLD names include .com, .edu, .gov, .net, and .org. The TLD name can assist the consumer in identifying the source and potential motives of each site. The TLD .gov denotes a government site. This TLD can be the source of good health information. Sites that are sponsored by the federal government:

> The U.S. Department of Health and Human Services (www.hhs.gov)
> The FDA (www.fda.gov)
> The National Institutes of Health (www.nih.gov)
> The Centers for Disease Control and Prevention (www.cdc.gov)
> The National Library of Medicine (www.nlm.nih.gov).

All the sites have updated information and are believed to be free of commercial bias.

The TLD .edu denotes an education site. This also is a very good source of health information. Sites that are run by universities or medical schools include Johns Hopkins University School of Medicine and the University of California–Berkeley hospital health system and other health care facility sites like the Mayo Clinic and Cleveland Clinic. These sites will present medical information directed at informing the consumer as well as describing particular areas of the medical center that will address these certain problems.

Organizations are denoted by the TLD .org. They also are good sources of health information. These sites are maintained by not-for-profit groups whose focus is research and teaching the public about specific diseases or conditions.

Cancer specific sites include:

American Cancer Society (http://cancer.org)
The National Cancer Institute (http://cancer.gov)
The Association of Cancer Online Resources (http://acor.org)
Cancer Care (http://cancercare.org)

Heart disease organizations include:

The American Heart Association (http://americanheart.org)
The National Heart, Lung, and Blood Institute (http://www.nhlbi.nih.gov)
The Congenital Heart Information Network (http://tchin.org)

Organizational sites for diabetes include:

The American Diabetes Association (http://diabetes.org)
The National Diabetes Education Program (http://ndep.nih.gov)
The Joslin Diabetes Center (http://www.joslin.harvard.edu)
Diabetes Monitor (http://diabetesmonitor.com)

Alzheimer's disease organizational sites include:

The Alzheimer's Association (http://alz.org)
The Fisher Center for Alzheimer's Research Foundation (http://alzinfo.org)

The TLD .com is short for "commercial," which pertains to a business or a product. These sites at times can be informative and impressive. It is always best to keep in mind that commercial sites are also interested in selling products or services. These sites may supplement medical information but should be consulted after visiting the aforementioned sites.

Health Sites

Certain sites contain information on a number of medical topics and serve as very good initial sites to visit to commence education regarding a particular diagnosis.

Medlineplus.gov: Sponsored by the National Institutes of Health and managed by the NLM, MedlinePlus provides information on more than 900 diseases and conditions in its "Health Topics" section and links to other trusted resources.

MayoClinic.com: Owned by the Mayo Foundation for Medical Education and Research, this site is produced by more than 3,300 physicians, scientists, and researchers from the Mayo Clinic and provides in-depth, easy-to-understand information on hundreds of diseases and conditions, drugs and supplements, tests, and procedures.

Another good site for medical information is Healthfinder.gov. This site is sponsored by the Office of Disease Prevention and Health Promotion within the U.S. Department of Health and Human Services. The site is written for consumers and has recommendations for preventative care based on gender and age. In addition it has information on a number of health topics from A–Z.

False Claims

Snake oil salesmen have been around for centuries. These individuals may be easy to spot, and consumers are very aware of their tactics. Claims on the Internet may be harder to interpret. An Internet site may have impressive graphics or seem official or part of an organization. As mentioned before, TLDs with .com are a commercial site, and their intent more than likely is to promote or sell a product rather than provide unbiased information to the consumer.

Be aware when a product claims "One Product Does It All." The product may be promoted to help with heart disease, back pain, diabetes, and cancer. Those disease processes are entirely different from one another, and one medicine has not been found to treat all of them. The aforementioned diagnoses do have one thing in common: They are the most commonly diagnosed conditions in the United States. These products also are supported by personal testimonies, but remember this is not considered an adequate form of medical evidence.

The term *natural* is often associated with safe. This is not always the case. Natural products can certainly be dangerous. Botulinum is produced by bacteria naturally and can be fatal if ingested; rattlesnakes and their venom are also natural. If a product was a cure for a serious disease, it would be widely reported in the media. It would then be regularly prescribed by health professionals. The miracle product would not be found in a magazine or newspaper ad, late-night television show, or infomercial.

Quick fixes are also a concerning claim. Unfortunately, cancer cannot be eliminated in a few days with any product at this time. The cures will usually target the individuals with chronic pain or a diagnosis with limited medical treatments. The claims may also involve paranoid accusations in an attempt to gain one's support or belief in the product. Examples may include the following catch phrase: "Get the all-natural cure the drug companies are trying to hide." This claim suggests that health care providers and legitimate manufacturers are partnering to promote prescribing their products for a mutual financial gain.

NEED TO KNOW

Consumers (patients) need to be somewhat cautious in regard to chat rooms. Chat rooms can at times be helpful in obtaining a better understanding of a disease, illness, or sickness. The understanding can come from one person relating his or her experiences of a particular disease. These experiences can help other patients by providing them with a better understanding of the disease and can give them a better understanding of what symptoms and potential course of the disease to expect. Caution is advised when it comes to treatments. Patients may tout various treatments or health care providers who provided miraculous cures. These may be individuals who truly do not have the disease providing false information in an attempt to sell a product or influence a potentially desperate (hoping to find a cure/treatment) patient to a certain health care provider.

References

1. Hartzband, P., & Groopman, J. (2010). Untangling the web—patients, doctors, and the Internet. *New England Journal of Medicine, 362,* 1063–1066.
2. Tang, H., & Ng, J. H. K. (2006). Googling for a diagnosis—use of Google as a diagnostic aid: Internet based study. *BMJ, 333,* 1143–1145.

35

Medical Myths

Objective

▸ Review of 10 common medical myths

Urban Legend

An urban legend, as defined by *Oxford Dictionary* is "a humorous or horrific story or piece of information circulated as though true, especially one purporting to involve someone vaguely related or known to the teller."[1] A classic example of an urban legend is Mikey from LIFE cereal fame. Mikey was a child actor who starred in a television ad for LIFE cereal. Legend has it that Mikey died after consuming Pop Rocks® (candy) and drinking carbonated soda. When these two products are combined, they form significant amounts of CO_2 (carbon dioxide) gas. Not enough to kill a human being, let alone Mikey, but enough to cause significant belching. But the urban myth has perpetuated; just ask a Generation X individual and they will tell you what they were told.

This chapter will consist of stating the myth and then information to either prove or debunk them.

> *Physicians with poor bedside manners are superior when it comes to care and knowledge.*

This statement and belief is false. Rude physicians are rude physicians. The public perception is that if physicians are blunt or terse in their interaction, they are very busy. If they are very busy, they must be good (since so many patients are scheduled to see them). The physician's interaction is now being reported in various patient satisfaction surveys, which are available for public review. The days of the rude physician are numbered.

Sit-ups are a good exercise to get a flat stomach.

This statement is false. In a small randomized controlled trial in 1983, two groups were compared; one group did daily sit-up exercises while the control group did none. The total number of sit-ups done was 5,004. After 27 days, fat biopsies were taken from the abdomen, subscapular, and gluteal sites. Fat samples showed no significant differences in the rate of change (pre to post) in cell diameter between sites for the experimental and control groups ($p > .05$). Body weight, total body fat (underwater weighing), and fatfolds and girths remained unaltered. The results demonstrate that the conventional sit-up exercise does not preferentially reduce adipose cell size or subcutaneous fat thickness in the abdominal region to a greater extent compared to other adipose sites.[2]

Other studies have shown the sit-up to create up to 3000N of force (674 pounds) in the low back (lumbar) region.[3] Such increases in intradiscal pressure can help to promote and exacerbate preexisting disc conditions. Another study conducted on new agent trainees of the FBI showed that 46.8% of injuries during physical fitness training were caused by sit-ups.[4] Lastly, there has been a case report that describes the rupturing of an ovarian cyst following a series of 12 sit-ups.[5]

You will get arthritis if you crack your knuckles.

This belief is false and possibly started by parents who found their children who cracked their knuckles annoying. There is no evidence that knuckle cracking causes arthritis. Habitual knuckle cracking in children has been considered a cause of arthritis. A survey of a geriatric patient population with a history of knuckle cracking failed to show a correlation between knuckle cracking and degenerative changes of the meta-carpal phalangeal joints.[6] When you crack your knuckles, you're causing the bones of the joint to pull apart. This pulling action then causes a gas bubble to form within the joint. The cracking or popping sound you hear is the breaking of the adhesive seal in the joint by the gas bubble.

If you don't work out, your muscles will turn into fat.

This statement is false. Muscles and fat are completely different tissues and components of the body. Different tissues do not turn into other tissues. People will add fat to their bodies if their intake of calories is greater than calories expenditure for the day. They will lose fat if they burn more calories than they take in for the day. For muscle tissue, people can gain muscle mass (hypertrophy) with exercise and can lose muscle mass with lack of strength training. Loss of muscle mass will also naturally occur with aging.

Thanksgiving dinner with turkey, which is loaded with tryptophan, will cause you to sleep.

Tryptophan is an amino acid. Amino acids are the building blocks for protein and muscles. We also know that tryptophan is involved in sleep and mood control and can cause drowsiness. Turkey does not contain a higher concentration of tryptophan than other meats, including chicken, pork, or beef. Turkey meat contains about 205mg/100gm.[7] Other foods, including fish, contain a higher concentration of tryptophan. Eggs contain a slighter lower concentration, at 180mg/100gm, but one will promote starting their day off with eggs for energy. The sleepiness following the Thanksgiving dinner may be related to the changes in blood flow. Following such a meal, there will be increased blood flow to the digestive tract and reduced flow to the brain. In addition, accompanying alcohol may also play a role.

Sugar will cause hyperactivity in kids.

This is also false, with a number of studies showing no effect exists. One study tested 35 5- to 7-year-old boys reported by their mothers to be behaviorally sugar sensitive, and their mothers. The mothers in the experimental group were told their children had received a large dose of sugar, whereas in the control condition mothers were told their sons received a placebo; all children actually received the placebo (aspartame). Mothers and sons were videotaped while interacting together. Review of the interactions showed the mothers who thought their sons had received the sugar exercised more control by maintaining physical closeness, as well as showing trends to criticize, look at, and talk to their sons more than did control mothers.[8] Another study looked at boys with attention deficit disorder (ADD) and found that sugar does not adversely affect the behavior or learning of ADD boys.[9] High sugar intake has been linked to causing other medical problems including obesity and diabetes. The myth has likely persisted because if a young child is told that ingesting sugar will cause increased activity, they may believe it to be true and exhibit behavior to support the belief. Additionally, sugar is often given at times when the rules are loosened and there are lots of other kids present at birthday parties and holidays, which can lead to an increased baseline of excitement and activity.

You are Ok eating food off the floor if you adhere to the 5-second rule.

This practice is certainly not advised. This statement actually depends on where the food lands, more so than how long the food is on the floor. If the food lands in an area with contamination, it will likely get contaminated. This hypothesis was recently examined. Examiners used four different surfaces (stainless steel, ceramic tile, wood, and carpet), four different foods (watermelon, bread, bread with butter, and gummy candy), four different contact times (<1, 5, 30, and 300 seconds), and two bacterial preparation methods. They found the longer contact times result in more transfer, and the nature of the food and the surface are of equal or greater importance. Some transfer takes place instantaneously, at times of <1 second, disproving the 5-second rule.[10] Additional testing found over 99% of bacterial cells were transferred from a tile floor to a piece of bologna after 5 seconds of bologna exposure to tile as well as noting the bacteria *Salmonella typhimurium* can survive up to 4 weeks on dry surfaces.[11]

Measles, mumps, and rubella (MMR) vaccination has been scientifically shown to be a contributing factor to autism.

This myth was started in 1998 by an article in the journal *Lancet* by Dr. Andrew Wakefield and colleagues.[12] In the study, the parents of eight autistic children reported the onset of autistic symptoms following an MMR vaccination. The authors concluded that "possible environmental triggers" (MMR vaccine) were associated with the onset of both the gastrointestinal disease and developmental regression. Correlation was quickly confused with causation. Twelve years after publishing the paper, *The Lancet* retracted the paper. The *BMJ* said that it is now clear that several elements of the paper are incorrect. Britain's General Medical Council ruled in January 2017, that the children that Wakefield studied were carefully selected and some of Wakefield's research was funded by lawyers acting for parents who were involved in lawsuits against vaccine manufacturers.[13] Wakefield was found to have acted unethically as he performed invasive tests on the children involved in the study. The effect of the initial paper reduced immunization rates, which has led to a certain increase of the rates of measles, mumps, and rubella.

Since the 1998 study, many studies such as a 2002 study in the *New England Journal of Medicine* of 530,000 children have found nothing to suggest that vaccinations increase the risk of becoming autistic.[14] Unfortunately, the erroneous study has wasted significant time and funding to prove multiple times that the MMR vaccinations does not cause the condition.

Hot tubs do not affect a male's fertility.

Hot tubs can affect a male's fertility.[15] Elevated water temperatures can affect spermatogenesis, or the process of sperm formation. Men who are actively trying to reproduce should avoid temperatures greater than 100 degrees. The sperm are contained in the testicles in males. The testicles, being temperature sensitive, are contained outside of the body. They are housed in the scrotum, a sac that hangs in the genital region of males. The scrotum will react to differences in temperatures, thickening and retracting with cooler temperatures in an attempt to raise the internal temperature of the scrotal sac by being closer to the body. The scrotal skin will thin and become looser, allowing the testicles to hang further from the body on warm days, cooling its internal temperatures. It can take up to 6 months to recover normal sperm parameters, which include sperm count, movement, shape, and structure.

You can catch a cold from the cold weather in the winter.

There is no truth to this myth. A classic study published in 1968 in *the New England Journal of Medicine* showed what happens when researchers exposed people to the rhinovirus (common cause of the common cold) in different environmental conditions. The conditions included a 4°C room and 32°C bath water. The study demonstrated no effect of exposure to cold on host resistance to rhinovirus infection and illness that could account for the commonly held belief that exposure to cold influences or causes common colds.[15] It has been postulated that the common cold is more frequently observed during the winter months because people stay indoors more. Staying indoors increases the likelihood of closer contact with more people, thus increasing the chances of spreading and contacting the virus.

NEED TO KNOW

Beer before liquor never sicker, but liquor before beer in the clear.
This is a bit of advice that is passed on to college students. Is it true? No, alcohol is alcohol. The determining factor is the blood alcohol concentration (BAC). It is the BAC that will determine the effects on the body. The alcohol content of beer is lower than liquor's alcohol content. If one drinks the same number of beers and liquor drinks, the total alcohol concentration or BAC will be the same regardless of the order.

References

1. "art, n.1." *OED Online.* Oxford University Press, June 2017. Web. 30 October 2017.
2. Chang, Y. T., & Lin, J. Y. (2009). Intraperitoneal rupture of mature cystic ovarian teratoma secondary to sit-ups. *Journal of the Formosan Medical Association, 108*(2), 173–175. doi:10.1016/S0929-6646(09)60049-8
3. Dawson, P., Han, I., Cox, M., Black, C., & Simmons, L. (2007). Residence time and food contact time effects on transfer of Salmonella typhimurium from tile, wood and carpet: Testing the five-second rule. *Journal of Applied Microbiology, 102*(4), 945–953.
4. Douglas, R. G., Jr., Lindgren, K. M., & Couch, R. B. (1968). Exposure to cold environment and rhinovirus common cold—failure to demonstrate effect. *New England Journal of Medicine, 279,* 742–747.
5. Eggertson, L. (2010). Lancet retracts 12-year-old article linking autism to MMR vaccines. *Canadian Medical Association Journal, 182,* 4E199–E200.

6. Harada, T., Hirotani, M., Maeda, M., Nomura, H., & Takeuchi, H. (2007). Correlation between breakfast tryptophan content and morningness-eveningness in Japanese infants and students aged 0–15 yrs. *Journal of Physiological Anthropology, 26*(2), 201–207.

7. Hoover, D. W. R. (1994). Effects of sugar ingestion expectancies on mother-child interactions. *Journal of Abnormal Child Psychology, 22*(4), 501–515.

8. Katch, F. I., Priscilla, M., Clarkson, P. M., Kroll, W., McBride, T., & Wilcox, A. (1984). Effects of sit up exercise training on adipose cell size and adiposity. *Research Quarterly for Exercize and Sport, 3,* 242–247.

9. Knapik, J. J., Spiess, A., Swedler, D. et al. (2011). Retrospective examination of injuries and physical fitness during Federal Bureau of Investigation new agent training. *Journal of Occupational Medicine and Toxicoogy, 6,* 26. doi:10.1186/1745-6673-6-26

10. Madsen, K. M., Hviid, A., Vestergaard, M. et al. (2002). A population-based study of measles, mumps, and rubella vaccination and autism. *New England Journal of Medicine, 347*(19), 1477–1482.

11. McGill, S. M. (1995). The mechanics of torso flexion: Situps and standing dynamic flexion manoeuvres. *Clinical Biomechanics, 10*(4), 184–192.

12. Milich, R., & Pelham, W. E. (1986). Effects of sugar ingestion on the classroom and playgroup behavior of attention deficit disordered boys. *Journal of Consulting and Clinical Psychology, 54*(5), 714–718. Retrieved from http://dx.doi.org/10.1037/0022-006X.54.5.714

13. Miranda, R. C., & Schaffner, D. W. (2016). Longer contact times increase cross-contamination of *Enterobacter aerogenes from* surfaces to food. *Applied and Environmental Microbiology, 82*(21), 6490–6496.

14. Shefi, S., Tarapore, P. E., Walsh, T. J., Croughan, M., & Turek, P. J. (2007). Wet heat exposure: A potentially reversible cause of low semen quality in infertile men. *International Brazilian Journal of Urology, 33*(1). Retrieved from http://dx.doi.org/10.1590/S1677-55382007000100008

15. Swezey, R. L., & Swezey, S. E. (1975). The consequences of habitual knuckle cracking. *Western Journal of Medicine, 122*(5), 377–379.

16. Wakefield, A. J., Murch, S. H., Anthony, A. et al. (1998). Ileal-lymphoid-nodular hyperplasia, non-specific colitis, and pervasive developmental disorder in children. *Lancet, 351*(9103), 637–641.

International Travel

Objectives

▸ Basic understanding of common medical concerns for the traveler
▸ Knowledge of where to find timely travel medical information and treatments

International Travel

When it comes to traveling internationally, which of the following best describes your approach to travel? I take my passport, I visit my PCP prior to travel, or I plan my trip with medications, insurance, and a list of medical facilities for the countries in which I travel. One's preparation prior to travel can occasionally pay off in a big way. Most consumers may not consider or adequately prepare for potential medical problems.

Medical Insurance

Medicare generally does not provide for medical care or coverage in a foreign country. There are three exceptions to this rule, as noted by Medicare. The first one occurs when you are in the United States when you have a medical emergency, and the foreign hospital is closer than the nearest U.S. hospital that can treat your illness or injury. The second exception is when you are traveling through Canada by the most direct route between Alaska and another state when a medical emergency occurs. The Canadian hospital is closer than the nearest U.S. hospital, and coverage may be provided for care in the Canadian hospital after review by Medicare. The final exception occurs when you live in the United States and the foreign hospital is closer to your home than the nearest U.S. hospital that can treat your medical condition, regardless of whether it's an emergency.

Certain Medigap plans may cover international travel. According to Medicare, your Medigap policy may offer additional coverage for health care services or supplies that you get outside the U.S. Standard Medigap plans C, D, F, G, M, and

TABLE 36.1   TYPES OF TRAVEL INSURANCE

Type	Coverage
Travel insurance	Baggage, flight cancellations
Travel medical insurance	Foreign medical care
Medical evacuation insurance	Air ambulance or medical evacuation

Source: U.S. Department of State, Bureau of Consular Affairs.[1]

N provide foreign travel emergency health care coverage when you travel outside the United States. Plans E, H, I, and J are no longer for sale, but if you bought one before June 1, 2010, you may keep it. All of these plans also provide foreign travel emergency health care coverage when you travel outside the United States. The coverage is provided as long as the medical care starts within 60 days of leaving the United States.

There are three options regarding travel insurance. Travel Insurance is the type of coverage that covers your financial investment in your trip. It will cover lost baggage and cancelled flights. It is not medical insurance and does not cover medical costs. Travel Medical Insurance may be purchased and it will cover foreign medical treatment and care. The last type of insurance is Medical Evacuation Services. This insurance will provide coverage for air ambulance, medical evacuation or medical escort service coverage for overseas travelers. The website travelstate.gov has a listing of U.S.-based companies that sell travel and medical insurance. As with any insurance product it is best to fully understand what is covered and to what degree. The different insurance types are outlined in Table 36.1.

Deep Venous Thrombosis

Deep venous thrombosis (DVT) is a medical emergency that can be associated with travel. DVT is a blood clot that will traditionally occur in the leg(s). The clot may form in one of the large veins of the leg. The concern is if the clot suddenly separates from the vein, it can then end up in the lung. The clot can then obstruct the flow of blood necessary for oxygenation. If the clot is large enough it can be fatal. The individual may experience the sudden onset of chest pain associated with dyspnea (difficulty breathing).

Risk factors for the development of a DVT include a prior history of a blood clot. Another risk factor includes a family history of a blood clot, meaning a close family member has had a blood clot in the past. Other risk factors also include recent surgery, trauma to the leg and inactivity. Traveling in an airplane for hours with little to no movement of the legs is such an example of inactivity. Additional risk factors include oral contraception, pregnancy and smoking. See Table 36.2 for a list of risk factors.

The symptoms that a patient may experience with a DVT can vary. Some patients may experience little to no symptoms. Others may develop leg pain, increased warmth of the leg, and leg swelling. The calf's circumference can be measured at its largest girth and then compared side to side; if a greater than 2-centimeter difference is present, this may suggest a blood clot. The blood clot can be diagnosed in the legs with a Doppler study (ultrasound study examining the flow of blood through the area of concern). The treatment for a DVT is medications known as blood thinners. They are usually initiated via injections and then converted to oral (take by mouth) medications.

DVT prevention may include getting up occasionally and walking around the plane. One may also wish to exercise the calf muscles and stretch the legs while sitting. Selecting an aisle seat when possible may also help with leg stretching and movement.

Motion Sickness

Motion sickness occurs while riding in a car, bus or ship. It can occasionally occur with airplane travel. The travel will cause nausea and potential vomiting. For individuals who experience motion sickness the effects may be minimized by sitting in the front seat of the car or in front of a bus. Sitting at the level of the wing of an airplane may also help. For cruises, it is frequently recommended to get a central cabin, where there is less vertical motion. Medications, both over the counter and prescriptions (prescribed by a health care provider), can be very effective. Other types of effective treatment include mint, ginger, or sucking on a piece of candy.

Altitude Illness

Altitude illness occurs when one travels to a higher altitude and continues to ascend. This can occur with travel to foreign countries and the goal of hiking the

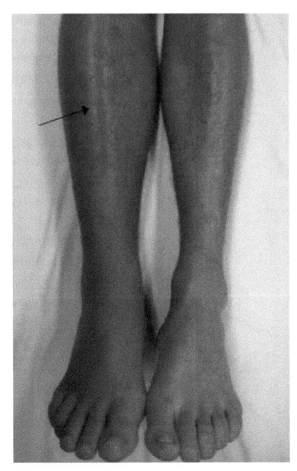

FIGURE 36.1 Deep Venous Thrombosis Patient with a DVT of the right leg.

TABLE 36.2 RISK FACTORS FOR A DVT

Prior history of a blood clot

Relative or family member with a blood clot history

Recent surgery

Leg or lower extremity trauma

Oral contraception

Smoking

Pregnancy

Prolonged inactivity (during an airplane trip)

mountains. The mountain ranges can include the Alps, Andes, or Himalayans. Altitudes of greater than 9,000 feet can present problems. If you plan to travel to a higher altitude and sleep there, you can get sick if you don't ascend gradually. It is recommended to start the trip at a level of 8,000 to 9,000 feet, by spending a few days at that level. One should not ascend greater than 1,600 feet per day. Many high-altitude destinations are remote. They lack access to medical care, so it is very important to focus on prevention rather than treatment or emergency care.

The symptoms of altitude illness are similar to those of a hangover. They include a headache, feeling tired, lack of appetite, nausea, and vomiting. For individuals experiencing these symptoms, it is very important not to ascend any further until the symptoms remit.

A person whose symptoms are getting worse while resting at the same altitude must descend or risk serious illness or possible death.

Prevention of altitude illness is the main focus. The medication acetazolamide is used to prevent or treat altitude illness. The medication can reduce pressures and help to rid the body of excess fluid. The medication is taken as a pill twice a day. It can be prescribed by your health care provider and taken with you on your trip.

Travelers' Diarrhea

Travelers' diarrhea is the most common travel-related illness. It can occur anywhere, but the highest-risk destinations are in most of Asia as well as the Middle East, Africa, Mexico, and Central and South America. In otherwise healthy adults, diarrhea is rarely serious or life-threatening, but it can certainly make for an unpleasant trip. There are a number of steps the traveler can take to avoid diarrhea on their trip.

The initial approach to travelers' diarrhea should be on prevention. It may be prudent to choose foods and beverages carefully to lower your risk of diarrhea. Eating only food that is cooked and served hot is preferred to eating raw fruits or vegetables. If consuming raw fruits and vegetables, washing them in clean water may reduce the risks. Drinking water or beverages from factory-sealed containers may be necessary. One should also avoid ice, as the source of the ice is likely the same as the tap water.

The likelihood of the diarrhea is reduced with frequent and proper washing of hands. It is important to wash your hands often with soap and water, or use an alcohol-based sanitizer especially after using the bathroom and before eating.

Treatment focuses on fluid replacement, antibiotics, and mediations to address the symptoms. People with diarrhea should drink lots of fluids to stay hydrated. Oral rehydration solutions available in pharmacies in developing countries can be used for fluid replacement. Alcohol should be avoided for fluid replacement, as it can promote dehydration. Alcohol has diuretic (promotes loss of fluid through urination) properties.

It blocks the action of antidiuretic hormone (ADH), which works to save water and fluid for the body.

Antibiotics can treat the diarrhea that are caused by bacteria. Many travelers carry antibiotics with them so they can treat diarrhea early if they start to get sick. The antibiotics can be obtained by visiting your health care provider prior to your international trip. Other treatments include a number of OTC drugs. Several drugs, such as Lomotil or Imodium, can be bought over the counter to treat the symptoms of diarrhea. These drugs decrease the frequency and urgency of needing to use the bathroom.

Additional Information

Additional information can be found on the CDC website. The information on the website is updated regularly. The site allows one to search a particular country and they will receive a list of recommended immunizations to obtain as well as medication recommendations.

Another resource is the CDC's TravWell app. This app can be downloaded to one's smart phone and is invaluable for international travel. The app will help you plan international travel. The app will provide information regarding destination-specific vaccine recommendations, a checklist of what you need to do to prepare for travel, and a customizable healthy travel packing list. The app also lets you store travel documents, keep a record of your medications and immunizations, and set reminders to get vaccine booster doses or take medicines while you're traveling. It also provides emergency services phone numbers for every destination and lists medical facilities for the countries on one's itinerary.

NEED TO KNOW

Can I Eat This?

When traveling, one wants to enjoy the local cuisine but not ruin the trip with a case of Montezuma's revenge, Delhi belly, or traveler's diarrhea. The CDC has an app available for international travel to address these concerns. To help prevent traveler's diarrhea, one can download the CDC's *Can I Eat This?* app. It allows users to select the country they are currently in and answer a few simple questions about what they are thinking about eating or drinking; the app will tell them whether it's likely to be safe or not.

Reference

1. https://travel.state.gov/content/passports/en/go/health/insurance-providers.html#insurance

Resources

Centers for Disease Control and Prevention—CDC sponsored traveler's page with information on travel, medicines and general advice: http://wwwnc.cdc.gov/travel/

U.S. Passports & International Travel—Department of the State site with information of the various types of travel insurance and valuable links for additional information: https://travel.state.gov/content/passports/en/go/health/insurance-providers.html

Figure Credits

Workers' Compensation

Objectives

- ▸ Basic understanding of the history of the workers' compensation system
- ▸ Understanding of the current workers' compensation systems in the United States
- ▸ Review of the process of being injured at work
- ▸ Knowledge of the physician–patient interaction in the compensation system

History

When people think of the workers' compensation system, they are very unlikely to think of a pirate. Yes, those pirates who sailed the seven seas robbing, looting, and committing other crimes. Pirates were a very well-organized group that realized there was an inherent risk to their occupation. They set up a compensation schedule as a reward to the potential sacrifice they may experience during their work.

In the mid-1600s, English privateer Captain Henry Morgan had a ship's constitution that provided for the "recompense and reward each one ought to have that is either wounded or maimed in his body, suffering the loss of any limb, by that voyage." The loss of a right arm was worth 600 pieces of eight; the left arm, 500; right leg, 500, left leg, 400; and so forth.[1] The pirates' compensation system was designed for different reasons, but it isn't that different from what exists today. For example, in the state of Connecticut, the difference in "value" between losing your right and left arms is roughly 7%, and it was estimated to be 6% for pirates on Captain Morgan's ships.[2]

The modern workers' compensation system has its origins in Europe. England and Germany both developed workers' compensation systems. Prussian chancellor Otto von Bismarck, under a degree of social unrest in Germany, created the Employer's Liability Law of 1871. This law required employees to pay part of the costs and called for highly centralized administration. Its coverage was broad, compulsory, and provided for nonprofit mutual employers' insurance funds.[3] In 1884, he established Workers' Accident Insurance. This program not only provided monetary benefits but medical and rehabilitation benefits as

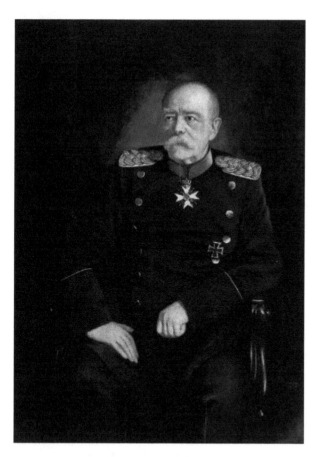

FIGURE 37.1 Portrait of Otto von Bismarck.

well. The centerpiece of von Bismarck's plan was the shielding of employers from civil lawsuits; thus the exclusive remedy doctrine was born.[4] Other European countries quickly imitated the German system.

The British workers' compensation law and system was very different than the German system. The English Poor Law was focused on the prevention of poverty and less with the prevention of disability.[5] The British system was an elective program and workers insurance could be obtained from private firms. This system was besieged with legal disputes from the beginning. Litigations focused on determining which jobs and industries were to be covered under the law.

In America, before a workers' compensation system was created; workers who were injured at work had to sue their employers for compensation for injuries. Initially, it was difficult to prove to a jury that the employer was at fault. In addition, the amounts awarded to injured workers varied greatly. With time, organized labor unions created pressure to pass laws placing less of a burden of the injured worker to prove fault with an accident. Juries became more sympathetic to the worker and the frequency and size of the monetary awards to injured workers increased. In response to this change, many companies incurred additional expenses in order to take out expensive employers' liability insurance policies. Reform was needed.

The first "workmen's" compensation law passed in the United States was the Federal Employer's Liability Act, which covered injured railroad workers. It was adopted in 1908 at the urging of President Theodore Roosevelt. The law placed the burden of proving that the railroad industry was at fault for the injury. President Roosevelt pointed out to congress that "the burden of an accident fell upon the helpless man, his wife and children" and that this was "an outrage."[6]

In 1911 Wisconsin was the first state to adopt the controversial "workmen's" compensation law. The law was known as the "great trade-off." The trade-off consisted of the following: The employer agreed to provide medical and wage replacement (indemnity) benefits; while the injured employee agreed to give up his or her right to sue the employer. This was believed to assist both sides reducing the costly worker's injury insurance the employer had to purchase, while providing the injured with benefits and not the burden to proving causality. Many states were quick to follow passing workers' compensation laws. The laws vary state to state. By 1948 all the states had at least some form of "workman's" compensation in effect, including the territories of Alaska and Hawaii.

Workers' Compensation in the United States

Today in the United States, there are two compensation systems a federal system and state systems. The federal system falls under the Federal Employee's Compensation Act (FECA). According to the United States Department of Labor, FECA provides workers' compensation coverage to three million federal and postal workers. The coverage includes wage replacement, medical and vocational rehabilitation benefits for work-related injury and occupational disease. Included among the executive, legislative and judicial branch employees covered by FECA are civilian Defense workers, medical workers in Veterans' hospitals, and the 800,000 workers of the Postal Service, the country's largest civilian employer.

FECA is touted as a highly cost-effective self-insurance system. Overhead is low, and because the system is no adversarial, the Federal government avoids time-consuming and expensive litigation. Disputes under the FECA are resolved through informal conferences or formal reconsideration at the district office level, through administrative hearing, or review by the independent Employees' Compensation Appeals Board, whose decision is final. Thus, employers avoid high legal costs and time-consuming litigation.

The workers' compensation system administered at the state level is a much different system. It is a system well entrenched within the legal system. Legal confrontations about the nature of the injuries, their extent and recoveries are challenged in the courts. Money is spent by the employer's insurance companies to minimize financial awards to injured workers. State programs pay for less than one third of the total costs of occupational injuries. These costs then become the responsibility of the workers, their families, private medical insurance, and Medicare and Medicaid to absorb.[7] Ten times as many severely disabled occupational disease victims receive Social Security Disability Insurance (SSDI) or early retirement benefits than those who receive workers' compensation benefits.[8] Most of the costs associated with work injuries are not being truly covered by workers' compensation. The legal issues no longer focus on the employer causing the injury, but on the nature of the injuries. There have been proposals to change the workers' compensation model of occupational and environmental medicine to a public health model due to these issues and place a greater emphasis on worker outcomes and less on costs.[9-10]

Occupational Safety and Health Act

The 1877 passage of the Massachusetts factory inspection law was done to improve and protect the worker's health and safety at the workplace.[11] Many states then implemented safety inspection systems for additional protection of the workers. Eventually unions were able to pressure lawmakers for federal protections for workers. This pressure lead to the Occupational Safety and Health Act of 1970, better known as OSHA. Congress enacted OSHA as well as commissioned an investigation into state workers' compensation laws. The commission found that there were serious flaws to most of the states' workers' compensation laws. While this investigation led to the most drastic state-level workers' comp reform in its 60 year history, the commission rejected federal takeover, simply stating: federal takeover would substantially disrupt established administrative arrangements. As a result of this lack of federal involvement, the laws and regulations in the United States today still vary greatly from state to state.[12]

Work Injury

What is the process when a worker is injured at work? Typically when someone is injured at work they will need to follow their injured worker protocol. The protocols vary from work place to work place. One universal recommendation is to report any work injury in a timely fashion. Early documentation is key to having the injury be covered for workers' compensation benefits.

Most reporting of the injury is done to the worker's supervisor who will then follow the appropriate protocol for reporting. The protocol may involve filling out a work injury claim form or information sheet. Depending on the severity of the injury, the injured worker may be sent emergently to the hospital, an occupational physician, or an on-site nurse. It is important to document any suspected injury or problem that occurs at work. The new onset of back pain may not seem like a big deal, but over the course of a few hours or even days it can become a significant problem.

Injuries of a significant nature may be seen by a physician or other health care provider. The health care provider may be hired by the company or from a list of providers that are paneled with the injured worker's company. The physician will then examine the injured worker and determine a diagnosis. Following the evaluation focus then will turn to an appropriate treatment plan in terms of the injury and work status. The injured worker may be kept out of work secondary to their injury or they may be able to return to work at full duty or without certain restrictions.

The injured worker may recover without incidence or the problem may linger and become a chronic one. The regulations governing workers' compensation vary from state to state, but in the state of Pennsylvania, after 90 days the injured worker can see a physician of their choice. The injured worker may choose to do this if they are not progressing or wish to obtain another opinion. In some cases, the insurance company for the employer or the employer may assign a case manager to assist the injured worker with their injury and claim.

The case managers are typically nurses who have additional training. They are assigned to a case to help coordinate care for the injured worker. They will serve as a liaison between the injured worker, the employer, the insurance company and treating physicians or health care providers. For patients with prolonged recovery periods the insurance company may order an independent medical examination (IME). An IME is performed by a physician to provide an independent assessment of the injured worker. The physician may specialize in the area of medicine that is involved with the particular injury. Following the IME and after review of the medical records associated with the case, the physician will submit a report offering their assessment of the patient, their work injury, treatments to date and future treatments.

TABLE 37.1   PHYSICAL DEMANDS OF JOB LEVELS

As defined by the U.S. Department of Labor:

a) **Sedentary work.** Sedentary work involves lifting no more than 10 pounds at a time and occasionally lifting or carrying articles like docket files, ledgers, and small tools. Although a sedentary job is defined as one which involves sitting, a certain amount of walking and standing is often necessary in carrying out job duties. Jobs are sedentary if walking and standing are required occasionally and other sedentary criteria are met.

b) **Light work.** Light work involves lifting no more than 20 pounds at a time with frequent lifting or carrying of objects weighing up to 10 pounds. Even though the weight lifted may be very little, a job is in this category when it requires a good deal of walking or standing, or when it involves sitting most of the time with some pushing and pulling of arm or leg controls. To be considered capable of performing a full or wide range of light work, you must have the ability to do substantially all of these activities. If someone can do light work, we determine that he or she can also do sedentary work, unless there are additional limiting factors such as loss of fine dexterity or inability to sit for long periods of time.

c) **Medium work.** Medium work involves lifting no more than 50 pounds at a time with frequent lifting or carrying of objects weighing up to 25 pounds. If someone can do medium work, we determine that he or she can also do sedentary and light work.

d) **Heavy work.** Heavy work involves lifting no more than 100 pounds at a time with frequent lifting or carrying of objects weighing up to 50 pounds. If someone can do heavy work, we determine that he or she can also do medium, light, and sedentary work.

e) **Very heavy work.** Very heavy work involves lifting objects weighing more than 100 pounds at a time with frequent lifting or carrying of objects weighing 50 pounds or more. If someone can do very heavy work, we determine that he or she can also do heavy, medium, light and sedentary work.

Another potential assessment of the injured worker is known as a functional capacity evaluation (FCE). The FCE is typically performed by a physical or occupational therapist. The FCE will assess the injured worker's capacity to lift, carry objects and other possible physical demands of the job. The FCE will provide recommendations as to the anticipated level of the work the worker can perform, as defined in Table 37.1. The recommendations may be temporary or permanent and dependent on the particular injury.

Predictive Factors

Workers' compensation cases can invoke strong feelings in an injured worker. These feelings can range from anger to frustration to feelings of abandonment. Some workers may feel that the company they worked for such a long time is turning their back on them because of their injury. There are a number of factors that play a role in determining if an injured worker will likely return to their previous job.

The predictive factors have been extensively studied as to their influence regarding return to work. Among workers with back injuries requiring surgery for a lumbar disc problem, researchers found the greatest predictor for return to work (RTW) following the surgery was their preoperative work status. 91.8% of injured workers who were working just prior to their back surgery RTW compared to 26.2% on injured workers who were not working prior to their surgery.[13] In addition, high physical and psychological job demands and low supervisory support are each associated with about 20% lower RTW rates during all disability phases. High job control, especially control over work and rest periods, is associated with over 30% higher RTW rates starting 30 days after injury.[14] Having low psychological job demands, high coworker and supervisor support and being in a low-strain job were all predictive of being in work 3 months after the end of the RTW program.[15]

Less is known about predictors of duration of work disability (DOD). One study found that the DOD increases with the time spent bending and lifting or pushing or pulling heavy objects at work, but it is unrelated to sitting, standing, or vibration. Younger age, longer preinjury employment, less severe injuries, and a previous back injury predicted shorter disability.[16] It is safe to say the workers' compensation system is influenced by a number of factors. In some ways the system of workers' compensation seemed a lot simpler in the days of the pirates.

References

1. Talty, S. (2007). *Empire of blue water: Captain Morgan's great pirate army.* New York: Crown Publishing.

2. Clark, P. (2011). The rich history of worker's compensation. *Business Insurance Quotes.* Retrieved from www.businessinsurance.org/the-rich-history-of-workers-compensation/#sthash.H5zr2J0U.dpuf

3. Gress, S., Gildemeister, S., & Wasem, J. (2004). The social transformation of American medicine: A comparative view from Germany. *Journal of Health Politics Policy Law, 29,* 679–699.

4. Guyton GP. A Brief History of Workers' Compensation. *The Iowa Orthopaedic Journal. 1999;* 19:106-110.

5. LaDou, J. (2011). The European influence on workers' compensation reform in the United States. *Environmental Health, 10,* 103. doi:10.1186/1476-069X-10-103

6. Florida Workers' Compensation Insurance. n.d. Home page. Retrieved from http://www.FloridaWC.com.

7. LaDou, J. (2010). Workers' compensation in the United States: Cost shifting and inequities in a dysfunctional system. *New Solutions, 20,* 291–302.

8. Reville, R. T., & Schoeni, R. F. (2004). The fraction of disability caused at work. *Social Security Bulletin, 65,* 31–37.

9. LaDou, J. (2006). Occupational and environmental medicine in the United States: A proposal to abolish workers' compensation and reestablish the public health model. *International Journal of Occupational and Environmental Health, 12*(2), 154–168.

10. Boden, L. I. (1995). Workers' compensation in the United States: High costs, low benefits. *Annual Review of Public Health, 16,* 189–218.

11. Asher, R. (2014). Organized labor and the origins of the Occupational Safety and Health Act. *New Solutions, 24*(3), 279–301. doi:10.2190/NS.24.3.d

12. Clark, P. (2011). The rich history of worker's compensation. *Business Insurance Quotes.* Retrieved from www.businessinsurance.org/the-rich-history-of-workers-compensation/#sthash.H5zr2J0U.dpuf

13. Than, K. D., Curran, J. N., Resnick, D. K., Shaffrey, C. I., Ghogawala, Z., & Mummaneni, P. V. (2016). How to predict return to work after lumbar discectomy: Answers from the NeuroPoint-SD registry. *Journal of Neurosurgery. Spine, 25*(2), 181–186. doi:10.3171/2015.10.SPINE15455

14. Krause, N., Dasinger, L. K., Deegan, L. J., Rudolph, L., & Brand, R. J. (2001). Psychosocial job factors and return-to-work after compensated low back injury: A disability phase-specific analysis. *American Journal of Industrial Medicine, 40*(4), 374–392.

15. Haveraaen, L. A., Skarpaas, L. S., Berg, J. E., & Aas, R. W. (2016). Do psychological job demands, decision control and social support predict return to work three months after a return-to-work (RTW) programme? The rapid-RTW cohort study. *Work, 53*(1), 61–71.
16. Dasinger, L. K., Krause, N., Deegan, L. J., Brand, R. J., & Rudolph, L. (2000). Physical workplace factors and return to work after compensated low back injury: A disability phase-specific analysis. *Journal of Occupational and Environmental Medicine, 42*(3), 323–333.

Resource

U.S. Department of Labor—Department of Labor site with specific information regarding compensation programs and rules governing them: https://www.dol.gov/general/topic/workcomp

Figure Credit

Fig. 37.1: Source: https://commons.wikimedia.org/wiki/File:Portrait_Bismarck_1894.jpg.

Long-Term Care

Objectives

- ▸ Basic understanding of what long-term care encompasses
- ▸ Review of long-term insurance
- ▸ Discussion of the different levels and costs associated with long-term care

Long-Term Care

Long-term care refers to a number of services and supports one may need to meet their personal care needs. Most long-term care is not true medical care, but rather assistance with the basic personal tasks of everyday life, sometimes called Activities of Daily Living (ADLs). ADLs may include bathing, dressing, using the toilet, transfers, and eating. These are skills that most take for granted but that can be a challenge in elderly individuals with underlying medical problems, which may include arthritis, stroke, or memory deficits (dementia).

Instrumental activities of daily living (IADLs) refer to activities that are necessary to managing a household. These may include housework, managing money, taking medication, meal preparation, and shopping. The U.S. Department of Health and Human Services (HHS) estimates that 70% of Americans older than 65 will require some level of long-term care. What factors play a role in determining who is more likely to require long-term care? One factor is age. As one ages, the likelihood of requiring care increases. In the United States the numbers of individuals receiving long-term care under the age of 65 is 3.6 million and above the age of 65 is 6 million.[1] Gender also plays a role; women have about a 5-year greater life expectancy than men and are more likely to be alone at home. Governmental statistics show that women need care longer on average (3.7 years) than men (2.2 years). If you live alone, you're more likely to need paid care than if you're married or living with someone.

Caregivers

Long-term care typically involves assistance with ADLs and IADLs, and for the most part this is not specialized medical care. The HHS estimates that about 80% of care at home is provided by unpaid caregivers who spend about spend 20 hours a week giving care. More than half (58%) have intensive caregiving responsibilities that may include assisting with a personal care activity, such as bathing or feeding. Caregivers are typically a family member or a friend. In the majority of cases, most adults may be able to live at home for many years with a combination of support from family, friends, and paid caregivers. When the care of an individual exceeds what can be provided in the home, there are a wide array of services, centers, and programs available.

Types of Long-Term Care

The different levels of long-term care are based on the needs of an individual and range from community support services to nursing facilities with 24-hour supervision. If specialized care is required, a nurse, home health or home care aide, and/or therapist may provide care at the house. The patient needs to qualify for *homebound* in order for some of these services to be covered. Medicare will consider a patient homebound if: You need the help of another person or medical equipment to leave your home, your doctor believes that your health or illness could get worse if you leave your home, or it is difficult for you to leave your home and you typically cannot do so. This type of care may be covered by Medicare on a short-term basis. Another type of care that can be given at home is hospice care for terminally ill people.

Community services are support services that can include adult day care, meal programs, senior centers, transportation, and other services. These can help people who are cared for at home and live with their families. For example, adult day care services provide a variety of health, social, and related support services in a protective setting during the day. The individual returns to the home in the evening, with supervision then being provided by perhaps an adult working child. This can help adults with impairments that affect memory and cognition (Alzheimer's disease or dementia). The services can also provide the caregiver with a much needed break or respite.

Other facility-based choices include assisted living, board and care homes, and continuing care retirement communities. Assisted living provides 24-hour supervision, assistance, meals, and healthcare services in a home-like setting. Services may include help with eating, bathing, dressing, toileting, taking medicine, transportation, laundry, and housekeeping. Social and recreational activities may also be available. Continuing care retirement communities (CCRCs) provide a full range of services and care based on what each resident needs over time. Care usually is provided in one of three main stages: independent living, assisted living, and skilled nursing.

Nursing homes offer care to people who cannot be cared for at home or in the community. They provide skilled nursing care, rehabilitation services, meals, activities, help with daily living, and supervision. Many nursing homes also offer temporary or periodic care.

Costs

The costs associated with the level of care also varies considerably. According to HHS, the costs can range from $21 per hour for a home health aide, $67 per day for adult day care center, and $229 per day for a private room in a nursing home. The costs are outlined in Table 38.1. The costs can also vary depending on the geographic region of the country one lives in.

How to Pay for Long-Term Care

Medicare does not typically pay or cover long-term care beyond a short period of time dependent on certain conditions being met. Medicare will pay for long-term care if one requires skilled services or rehabilitative care. Medicare will cover care in a nursing home for a maximum of 100 days and this usually follows an inpatient hospitalization for a new medical problem or diagnosis. The average Medicare covered stay is, on average, 22 days for this circumstance. Medicare does not pay for nonskilled assistance with Activities of Daily Living (ADL), which make up the majority of long-term care services. The patient will need to pay for long-term care services that are not covered by a public or private insurance program.

Medicaid does pay for the largest share of long-term care services. Medicaid is the federal insurance place for the poor that is administered at the state level. In order to

TABLE 38.1   LONG-TERM CARE COSTS

Level of Care	Cost
Homemaker services	$19 per hour
Home health aide	$21 per hour
Adult day care	$67 per day
Assisted living facility	$3,293 per month
Semiprivate room in nursing home	$6,235 per month
Private room in nursing home	$6,965 per month

Source: US Department of Health and Human Services (HHS).[2]

qualify for Medicaid your income and assets must be below a certain level. Congress passed the Deficit Reduction Act of 2005. This act has a look-back period of five years to examine an individual's assets to determine Medicaid eligibility. This act was passed to increase the look-back period from 3 years to 5 years. It was done to prevent fraud and limit the ability to allow financially wealthy individuals to transfer all of their assets to their children and then be eligible for free long-term nursing care.

Health insurance is either employer-sponsored or private health insurance, including health insurance plans, provides benefits and coverage similar to the coverage of Medicare, which is limited. It does cover long-term care, typically only for skilled, short-term, medically necessary care. There are an increasing number of private payment options including: long-term care insurance, reverse mortgages, life insurance options, and annuities that can fund long-term care costs.

Buying Long-Term Care Insurance

Long-term care insurance is private insurance and individuals with certain preexisting health conditions may not qualify for long-term insurance. For this reason it is recommended to purchase long-term care insurance well before you may need to use it.

One may not be eligible to purchase the insurance based on preexisting conditions. Some conditions include AIDS, any form of dementia, history of a stroke, and certain cancers. The conditions are listed in Table 38.2. Insurance companies also consider other health conditions when determining your eligibility. If you buy your long-term care insurance before you develop one of the health conditions listed above, then your policy will cover the care you need for that condition.

When purchasing the policy, it is best not to buy more than is needed. One may have adequate assets and enough income to pay a portion of their care costs and only need the policy to pay for the remainder. Also avoid buying too little insurance. The insurance policy may not be able to be changed once purchased, despite changes in one's health status.

It costs less to buy coverage when you are younger, so one can lock into a lower premium or rate, which may provide savings and longer coverage long term. The average age of people buying long-term care insurance today is about 60 years old. It is also important to know what specific types of long-term care are covered with the policy.

TABLE 38.2   LONG-TERM INSURANCE PREEXISTING CONDITIONS

Currently use long-term care services

Currently need help with activities of daily living

AIDS or AIDS-related complex

Alzheimer's disease or any form of dementia

Progressive neurological condition

Stroke or a history of strokes

Cancer or metastatic cancer

Home Care Services

Home care services are regulated at the state level and must be licensed. Consumers can check with their State health department to determine if the home care agency is licensed. Agencies may also be certified at the federal level by Medicare. Medicare will perform home health care agency inspections to assure they meet certain standards. The standards include federal health and safety requirements. Medicare will pay for services only if the agency is certified by Medicare.

The public can determine if the home health care agency is certified by Medicare, as well as reviewing its survey report. The consumer will need to call the Medicare Hotline at 1-800-633-4227 and ask for the Home Health Hotline for their State. One can then request a copy of the home health report from that hotline. In addition, one can determine if the agency has been accredited (awarded a seal of approval) by a group such as the Joint Commission on Accreditation of Healthcare Organizations (630-792-5800); http://www.jcaho.org) or the Community Health Accreditation Program (1-800-669-1656; http://www.chapinc.org).

Individuals can always contact their state consumer affairs office to see if any complaints have been filed against a particular home care agency. References from other families or patients who have worked with the agency can also be requested. Consumers may also request to see the certifications or licensure of the particular caregivers that will be coming into the house. Putting in the work on the front end may prevent problems or poor outcomes.

Nursing Home Factors to Consider

There are a number of factors to consider when choosing a nursing home for a loved one. Unfortunately, some decision-making capacity may be taken away simply by the cost of such facilities. An important factor to consider is when a senior spends down his or her life savings at a nursing home and then qualifies for Medicaid, will the nursing home accept Medicaid as a form of payment? The quality of the nursing home facility should also be a strong determining factor. The nursing home may be a new facility with high end common space areas and décor, but is this at the expense of proper staffing. While a 65-inch flat screen television can serve to provide a favorable impression during a tour of the facility, there are additional factors to consider. The state inspection report is available on Caregiverlist.com. and is based on an inspection once every 15 months.

An important factor to consider is the certified staff-to-resident ratio. Find out if the facility is able to provide one-to-one care if necessary. Staff longevity is another factor to inquire about. High staff turnover may be associated with staff feeling overwhelmed, overworked, and understaffed.

One can also inquire about activities that are available to the residents. Another clue may be the appearance of the residents; are they well-groomed and appropriately dressed? The cleanliness of the facility can also give an indication of the type of care provided. Are there strong odors of urine present? One may also consider the facilities policy on having pets visit. It may be helpful to consider what factors are important to the family and devise a checklist prior to visiting to allow for the factors to be properly assessed.

Review Public Information

As of January 2003, all Medicaid- and Medicare-certified nursing homes must publicly post the number of nursing staff they have on duty to care for residents on each daily shift. Licensed and unlicensed staff include registered nurses, licensed practical nurses, and certified nursing aides. Nursing homes must also make readily available the name and contact information for all state client advocacy agencies, the Medicaid fraud control unit, along with the results of the most recent state or federal survey.

NEED TO KNOW

Ombudsmen

An ombudsman is defined as an official appointed to investigate individuals' complaints against maladministration, especially that of public authorities. In Pennsylvania, ombudsmen will investigate and work to resolve complaints regarding long-term care services on behalf of consumers. They can serve as a resource regarding federal and state laws that govern these services.

References

1. Rogers, H. Komisar. Who Needs Long-Term Care? Fact sheet Georgetown University, Washington, DC (2003) https://longtermcare.acl.gov/costs-how-to-pay/costs-of-care.html

Resources

LongTermCare.gov—U.S. Department of Health and Human services site with specific page on the basics of long term care: https://longtermcare.acl.gov/the-basics/index.html

Medicare.gov—Webpage with information on long term care and links to assist with identifying appropriate care providers and facilities: https://www.medicare.gov/coverage/long-term-care.html

The Joint Commission—Webpage that outlines the role of the joint commission as well as links to determine a facilities current accreditation status: https://www.jointcommission.org/

Community Health Accreditation Partner—Homepage of an agency that works to accredit home health agencies and can serve as a resource in identifying these agencies: http://www.chapinc.org/what-we-do/chap-accreditation.aspx

39

Advance Directives and End-of-Life Issues

Terms

As Benjamin Franklin once said, "Our new Constitution is now established, everything seems to promise it will be durable; but, in this world, nothing is certain except death and taxes."[1] Death is part of the life process. The idea of death can be difficult to think about and potentially plan for. An advanced directive as defined by the National Cancer Institute is a legal document that allow you to spell out your decisions about end-of-life care ahead of time. The advance directive may include a living will and a durable power of attorney for health care. An advance directive is a legal document that goes into effect only if you are incapacitated and unable to speak for yourself.

A *living will* contains your instructions, including which treatments you want if you are dying or permanently unconscious. You can accept or refuse medical care. A *durable power of attorney* for health care is a legal document that names your health care proxy. Your proxy is someone you trust to make health decisions for you if you are unable to do so.

Advance care planning involves learning about the types of decisions that might need to be made ahead of time and then establishing an advance directive. Part of the process is to understand what is meant by artificial respirations, cardiopulmonary resuscitation (CPR), and nutritional support. Some patients simply respond with, "I don't want to be put on machines"; while this may be their decision, it is helpful to understand the different types of medical support available. Another important factor to remember is that individuals' advanced directives can be changed or modified, as per their wishes.

Cardiopulmonary Resuscitation

Cardiopulmonary resuscitation (CPR) refers to treatments that may be employed in an attempt to restore a normal heart rhythm; when an individual collapses secondary to problems of the heart. These problems may occur when the heart is not able to beat in a normal matter. The heart may be beating at an irregular very high rate or in an uncoordinated fashion (fibrillations). In either case, the heart output is not sufficient to sustain life and constitutes a medical emergency.

CPR was developed in an attempt to continue flow of blood from the heart to the body and to restore the heart rhythm. CPR typically involves performing chest compressions on the collapsed victim and analyzing the heart rhythm for possible defibrillations. Historically, CPR involved the rescuer breathing into the collapsed individual's mouth in an attempt to provide some oxygen into the person's lungs. This was then followed by chest compressions. The chest is compressed in an attempt to deliver blood from the heart to the other areas of the body. Recently, there has been more emphasis placed on chest compressions and less on mouth-to-mouth resuscitation.

The other aspect of CPR focuses on restoring the heart rhythm. This can be done with the use of an *automated external defibrillator* (AED). The AED is invaluable in potentially saving a person with a fatal heart arrhythmia (irregular beat). AEDs are identified by readily available signs. Their presence in public spaces, including arenas, gyms, and malls, has been increasing.

AEDs are very simple to use. Once the case is opened, the pads are to be placed on the collapsed victim, as shown on accompanying cartoons. Once the pads are placed on the chest, the machine is turned on. The machine will then verbalize what is occurring and what is going to occur. After the AED has analyzed the victim's heart rhythm, it

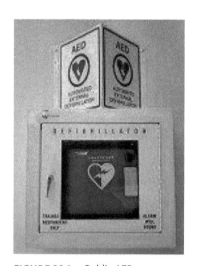

FIGURE 39.1   Public AED.

may advise delivering an electric shock. The shock is given the heart muscle in an attempt to restore the normal electrical conductivity and rhythm to the heart. The AED will then verbalize to "stand clear" as it delivers the shock. It will then analyze the heart to determine if the rhythm is changed. After analyzing the heart, the AED may advise continuing CPR (chest compressions) or another course of action.

Outcomes for CPR vary and have been studied for cardiac arrests that occur outside of the hospital with those that occur within the hospital. According to the AHA, there were 359,400 reported incidences of cardiac arrests in 2013 that occurred in public; bystander CPR was performed in 40.1% of those cases, with a survival rate of 9.5%. When a patient in the hospital suffers a cardiac arrest, is the outcome better? The reported survival to hospital discharge varies with the most common range being between 15% and 20%.[2] Research has shown that the sooner CPR can be started, the better the outcome. CPR has been found to be effective if started within 4 to 6 minutes from the time of the collapse and must be followed within 10 to 12 minutes of the collapse by advanced life support.[3]

Ventilator

A ventilator may be referred to as a breathing machine. This medical device will regulate breathing to ensure adequate oxygenation. The patient is connected to the machine with a tube. The tube connects the machine to the patient's trachea or windpipe. The ventilator will force oxygenated air into the lungs. The process of having a tube placed into the trachea is uncomfortable, and most patients will require sedation with medications while on the ventilator. If the patient is expected to be on the ventilator for more than a few days, a tracheotomy will be performed. This is a small tube that can be placed through the skin and directly into the trachea, bypassing the mouth. The tracheotomy allows for easy access into the trachea and bronchus. This access helps to allow for suctioning of lung secretions. If the patient's medical condition improves and they no longer require a ventilator, the tracheotomy tube can be fitted with a valve to permit speaking. The tube can also be plugged and if the patient tolerates the plugging the tube can be removed. The opening will be covered by a bandage and the opening will close on its own within a few days and does not require surgical closing.

Artificial Nutrition

If patients are unable to eat food safely, a feeding tube may be placed. Patients recovering from a stroke or a head injury may require a feeding tube to provide adequate nutrition during their recovery. The feeding tube will provide adequate nutrition. These measures can be helpful if one is recovering from an illness. Initially, the feeding tube is threaded through the nose down to the stomach. This type of tube is known as a nasogastric (NG) tube. The tube is named for the anatomy that it traverses, *naso-*, since it is inserted in the nose, and *gastric* referring to the stomach, the destination of the tube. If a feeding tube is needed for a number of days, a gastric tube can be placed. This is usually done by a gastroenterologist who surgically inserts the tube directly from the stomach and into the stomach. The tube provides easy access for nutrition, medications, and fluids.

If the tube is no longer needed, it can easily be removed. The opening for the tube will close on its own.

Artificial Hydration

When individuals are unable to drink water or swallow liquids, they can receive fluids via an IV route. The fluids and medications will be given via an IV, which involves placing a small plastic tube (catheter) into a vein. The IV is usually placed into a vein in the hand or arm (usually in the forearm area) to provide fluid when a person is unable to take in fluid. Medications can also be given via an IV route. The fluid is usually supplied in a clear bag and hung on a pole. It uses gravity to introduce the fluid into the body. The IVs placed into the arms need to be rotated and changed every few days to lower the risk of a skin infection.

Comfort Care

Comfort care is done to soothe and relieve suffering while staying in line with the patient's wishes. It may include managing shortness of breath, offering ice chips for dry mouth, placing limits on medical testing, providing medications for pain or anxiety, and providing emotional support. The emotional support may be in the form of spiritual and emotional counseling.

Hospice care is intended to provide comfort to you and your family during a life-threatening illness, rather than provide treatments to cure the illness. Hospice care does not imply no care and utilizes comfort care measures. It generally does not include additional diagnostic testing.

Palliative care differs from hospice care in that it is offered along with any medical treatments you might be receiving for a life-threatening illness. The tenets of both hospice and palliative care are to keep the patient comfortable. It is important to keep in mind that one can always move from hospice to palliative care if one wants to pursue treatments during an illness.

Living Will

A living will is a written document that helps you tell doctors how you want to be treated if you are dying or permanently unconscious and cannot make decisions about emergency treatments. The living will states in writing the patient's choices in regard to CPR, artificial ventilation, artificial nutrition, dialysis, and certain medications. A living will defines which of the procedures described an individual would want and which ones an individual would not want.

Durable Power of Attorney for Health Care

Durable power of attorney of health care is a legal document naming a health care proxy. A proxy is an individual appointed to make medical decisions for you at times when you might not be able to do so. The proxy should be familiar with your values and wishes. This means that he or she will be able to decide as you would when treatment decisions need to be made.

The proxy might be a family member, a friend, your lawyer, or someone with whom you know from your church. It's a good idea to also name an alternate proxy. It is especially important to have a detailed living will if one chooses not to name a proxy. The proxy can be given total authority over one's medical care or specific limitations. The decision to choose a proxy needs to be discussed over carefully with the prospective proxy to ensure they are comfortable with this responsibility.

Additional Advance Care

A do not resuscitate (DNR) order informs the medical staff in a hospital or nursing facility that you do not want them to try to return your heart to a normal rhythm if it stops or is in an unstable rhythm. Even though a living will might say CPR is not wanted, it is helpful to have a DNR order as part of your medical file if you go to a hospital. Posting a DNR next to your bed might avoid confusion in an emergency situation.

Organ and tissue donation can be considered as part of advance care. The donation allows organs or body parts from a generally healthy person who has died to be transplanted into patients who need them. Commonly, the heart, lungs, pancreas, kidneys, corneas, and liver are donated. Hospitals may at the time of death, ask the family of the deceased about organ donation.

Donating your body to science is another option. The body is generally donated for scientific study. The specific purpose can also be specified. The process involves contacting a local medical school, university or donation program for information on how to register for a planned donation for research.

After one has discussed their advanced planning wishes with their health care provider and determined their proxy, the next step is to fill out the necessary legal forms. Lawyers can help with this process, but are not required. Many states have their own advance directive forms. Your local Area Agency on Aging can help you locate the right forms. You can find your area agency phone number by calling the Eldercare Locator toll-free at 1-800-677-1116 or going online at http://www.eldercare.gov.

Copies of your advance directives should be given to your health care proxy, health care provider, and key family members. If you have to go to the hospital, give the staff there a copy to include in your records. It may be best to review your advance care planning decisions from time to time. You may wish to revise your preferences for care if your situation or your health changes.

What happens if you have no advance directive, the state where you live will assign someone to make medical decisions on your behalf? This will probably be your spouse, partner, your parents or children if they are adults. If you have no family members, the state will choose someone to represent your best interests.

Physician Order for Life-Sustaining Treatment

Some states make use of a physician order for life-sustaining treatment (POLST). This order is intended for people who have already been diagnosed with a serious illness. This form does not replace a patient's advance directives. It serves as doctor-ordered instructions to ensure that, in case of an emergency, you receive the treatment you prefer.

A POLST stays with you. If you are in a hospital or nursing home, the POLST is posted near your bed, where emergency personnel or other medical team members can easily find it. The doctor will fill out the form based on the contents of your directives, discussions with your doctor about the likely course of the illness, and your treatment preferences. These forms vary by state, but essentially a POLST enables your doctor to include details about what treatments not to use, under what conditions certain treatments can be used, how long treatments may be used, and when treatments should be withdrawn. The differences between a POLST and advance directives are described in Table 39.1.

TABLE 39.1   DIFFERENCES BETWEEN A POLST AND AN ADVANCE DIRECTIVE

	POLST	Advance directive
Population:	Sick, very ill	All adults
Time frame:	Current care	Future care
Who completes:	Physician	Patient
Form:	Medical orders	Advance directive

NEED TO KNOW

If you suffer a cardiac arrest in the United States, which city has the best survival rate? The answer is Seattle, Washington. According to King County EMS, someone who has a cardiac arrest in King County has a greater chance of survival than anyone else in the world. The survival rate for cardiac arrest in King County hit an all-time high of 62% in 2013.[1] By comparison, the cardiac survival rates in New York City, Chicago, and other urban areas have been recorded in the single digits.

Seattle is able to have this remarkable distinction for a number of reasons. The city has adopted high-performance CPR methods by emergency medical technicians in order to maximize oxygen circulation and increase survival chances. The county also utilizes telecommunications CPR, whereby 911 emergency personnel provide instant CPR instructions by phone. The city has prioritized the increasing public availability of AEDs. Local residents also have very high rates of CPR training. Lastly, Seattle supports a regional paramedic training program, funded by charitable contributions, that exceeds national standards for certification. There is emphasis at all levels to improve outcomes.

References

1. Franklin, Benjamin. Letter to Jean Baptiste Leroy, 1789. MS. Philadelphia, United States.
2. Sandroni, C., Nolan, J., Cavallaro, F., & Antonelli, M. (2007). In-hospital cardiac arrest: Incidence, prognosis and possible measures to improve survival. *Intensive Care Medicine, 33*(2), 237–245.
3. Cummins, R. O., Eisenberg, M. S., Hallstrom, A. P., Litwin, P. E. (1985). Survival of out-of-hospital cardiac arrest with early initiation of cardiopulmonary resuscitation. *American Journal of Emergency Medicine, 3*(2), 114–119.

Resources

Elder Care—U.S. Agency of aging sponsored site that allows for consumers to identify specific long term services for their particular location by entering their zip code: http://www.eldercare.gov

Figure Credit

40

Patient Satisfaction

Objectives

- ▸ Understanding of why there is an emphasis on patient satisfaction
- ▸ Review of the limitations of using patient satisfaction as an outcome metric
- ▸ Examples of patient satisfaction

History

There has recently been an emphasis by the CMS placed on patient satisfaction as this metric has been believed to reflect the quality of care received. Historically, health care providers have been paid by the fee for service principle. Fee for service is a method in which doctors and other health care providers are paid for each service performed. The more patients or procedures a provider does the more they are reimbursed.

Another reimbursement model is capitation. In capitation the health care provider is paid a set amount per person assigned to them. They are paid a set fee regardless of whether that person seeks treatment.

There has been a move toward the value-based purchasing payment model. This system rewards physicians, hospitals, medical groups, and other health care providers for meeting certain performance measures for quality and efficiency. It can also penalize health care providers for poor outcomes, medical errors, or increased costs.

Fee for Service

In the current fee-for-service model of reimbursing providers for health care, physicians and organizations have incentives to do more. The more tests you order, patients you see, procedures you do, the more money you will make. The financial risk with this model lies with the insurer or payer, as their costs can vary based on the services provided. One effect of this payment based on the volume model is enormous variation in rates of procedures and tests such as imaging and screening, done both on a local or regional level. Such variations raise questions as to why it costs more money to care for the same diagnosis in different parts of the same city, state, or country. According to The Dartmouth Atlas of Health Care, there is a 2.5-fold variation in Medicare spending nationally, even after adjusting for differences in local prices, age, race, and underlying health of the population. This geographic variation in spending is unwarranted. Increased spending does not show evidence of better health outcomes.

Capitation

The system of capitation places the financial risks on the health care providers and not on the insurers. The insurers will pay a fixed amount of money per year for each person (covered lives) in the plan. If the health care provider needs to provide services that exceed the cost they were reimbursed for the patient's care they will lose money and if they provide less care or services they will make money. The obvious concern with such a system is that it has the possibility of a financial disincentive for providing care.

Value-Based Purchasing

Value-based purchasing was created to address concerns of the fee for service and capitation models. This model is based on the value equation: Quality over Cost over Time. This system addresses patient concerns with appropriate, safety, and care with measureable results. For physicians, this model places a premium on employing evidence-based medicine and the patient's wishes and preferences. Evidence-based medicine refers to treatments that have been shown in the literature (medical journals and publications) to be effective and proven treatments.

Measurement is an important component of this model. This means that outcomes need to be measured and tracked. This information then allows for the public to review it and have a better understanding of the costs and outcomes of different treatments. Such information allows for better decision making for the public.

The CMS, hospitals, and insurance providers alike are striving to better define and measure quality of health care. They feel that a major component of quality of health care is patient satisfaction. The value-based purchasing system bases the reimbursements to providers on the patient's satisfaction. Satisfaction levels are felt to be influenced by the quality of care that is delivered. In this system, hospitals that provide a higher quality of care than their peers will receive reimbursement incentives, and hospitals that provide a lower quality of care will be penalized.

Quality of care is measured with two metrics: patient outcomes (70%) and patient satisfaction (30%).[1] With patient satisfaction scores now having a direct impact on the bottom line, the measure and management of patient satisfaction has become a top priority at health systems across the country. Because of the emphasis on patient satisfaction, more than half (54%) of health care executives say patient experience and satisfaction is one of their top three priorities.[2] Patient satisfaction carries the potential for both financial rewards and for financial penalties. The most commonly used measure of patient satisfaction is the Hospital Consumer Assessment of Healthcare Providers and Systems (HCAHPS).

HCAHPS

HCAHPS is a survey in which patients answer 32 questions to rate their inpatient hospital stay. The hospitals can either lose or gain a percentage of their Medicare payments based on the surveys. The CMS will increase the stakes over the next couple of years, with 2% of reimbursement dollars ultimately being at risk by fiscal year 2017. The metrics utilized to determine overall quality of care, will also adjust reducing the patient satisfaction component from 30% to 25%.

The HCAHPS survey was produced to provide a standardized survey instrument and data collection methodology for measuring patients' perspectives on hospital care. HCAHPS now serves as the national standard for collecting and publicly reporting the patient satisfaction data. According to the CMS, the HCAHPS survey has achieved its three goals.

The survey is designed to produce comparable data on the patient's perspective on care which allows objective and meaningful comparisons between hospitals on domains that are important to consumers. The public reporting of the survey results were designed to create incentives for hospitals to improve their quality of care. Public reporting has also served to enhance public accountability in health care by increasing the transparency of the quality of hospital care provided in return for the public investment.

The Survey

The HCAHPS survey contains 21 patient perspectives on care and patient rating items that encompass nine key topics: communication with doctors, communication with nurses, responsiveness of hospital staff, pain management, communication about medicines, discharge information, cleanliness of the hospital environment, quietness of the hospital environment, and transition of care. The survey also includes four screener questions and seven demographic items, which are used for adjusting the mix of patients across hospitals and for analytical purposes. The core of the survey contains 21 items that ask "how often" or whether patients experienced a critical aspect of hospital care, rather than whether they were "satisfied" with their care.

The survey can be administered via four routes: mail, telephone, mixed (mail with a follow-up telephone call) and active interactive voice response.

HCAHPS Timeline

In December 2005 the federal Office of Management and Budget gave its final approval for the national implementation of HCAHPS for public reporting purposes. The CMS implemented the HCAHPS Survey in October 2006, and the first public reporting of HCAHPS results occurred in March 2008. In 2013 the CMS added five new items to the HCAHPS Survey: three questions about the transition to post-hospital care, one about admission through the ER, and one about mental and emotional health.

HCAHPS is administered to a random sample of adult inpatients between 48 hours and 6 weeks after discharge. The survey is not restricted to Medicare patients. The hospitals are required to complete a minimum of 300 surveys over 12 months.

Public Reporting

The HCAHPS scores can be viewed online by consumers at: http://www.medicare.gov/hospitalcompare. This site allows consumers to compare HCAHPS scores at different hospitals. The scores are based on four consecutive quarters of patient surveys with the data being updated every 3 months. The CMS estimates that more than 8,400 patients complete the HCAHPS Survey every day.

HCAHPS Star Ratings

In April 2015 the CMS added HCAHPS Star Ratings to the Hospital Compare Web site. HCAHPS Star Ratings summarize the results for each HCAHPS measure and present it in a format that is easier to understand. The HCAHPS Star Ratings are also updated quarterly.

Hospitals must have at least 100 completed HCAHPS surveys over a four-quarter period and be eligible for public reporting of HCAHPS measures to receive HCAHPS Star Ratings. The HCAHPS Star Ratings can be found online at: http://www.hcahpsonline.org/StarRatings.aspx.

Emphasis on Outcomes

Patient satisfaction has been thought to improve outcomes, though this may not always be the case. Providers are aware of the questions that patients are asked. One provider tells the story that he scored very low with the "did your physician respect your privacy" survey question. He reports not changing his behavior in regard to patient privacy, but placing an added emphasis on it. For example, when seeing a patient in a semiprivate room he would always pull the curtain for privacy. After the survey results, he continued to pull the curtain for privacy, but would make a point to say, "I am now pulling the curtain for privacy." His scores for this question improved, but he did not change his behavior.

Another example of potential concern is the antibiotic dilemma. The physician correctly diagnoses the cause of an infection as viral (caused by a virus) in origin. Antibiotics are used to treat bacterial infections but are useless against viral infections. Overprescribing of antibiotics has led to the serious problem of bacterial resistance. The physician correctly does not prescribe antibiotics for the viral infection, but the child's mother is insistent on the antibiotics. Does the physician rightfully withhold the antibiotics and feel the wrath of low satisfaction scores or improperly prescribe the medications to appease the parent and likely receive high patient satisfaction scores? The same scenario can be repeated for narcotic medications, MRIs, and other treatments. The answers to these questions are certainly left to debate and questions the true value of this metric.

> **NEED TO KNOW**
>
> Cleveland Clinic is a nationally recognized hospital and health care center with an outstanding reputation. Its CEO, Dr. Cosgrove, noted that the clinic's patient satisfaction scores were lower than similar institutions. He contracted with an outside firm to conduct a study to see exactly what patients wanted. The results found the patient's top three concerns were: respect, good communication among staff, and happy employees during their stay. Respect is important to patients, as they want to be treated as individuals and not diseases or diagnoses. They desire providers to connect with them on a personal level and feel those providers will make fewer mistakes. The second was their concern with communication between caregivers. The perception is that a lack of communication between the physicians and nurses leads to substandard care. Lastly, patients want to see happy health care providers, as they feel the providers are more approachable. Patients tend not to ask the physicians as many questions if the physician is in a hurry or rushed.

References

1. Centers for Medicare & Medicaid Services. Medicare program; hospital inpatient prospective payment systems for acute care hospitals and the long-term care hospital prospective payment system and fiscal year 2013 rates; hospitals' resident caps for graduate medical education payment purposes; quality reporting requirements for specific providers and for ambulatory surgical centers. Final rule. *Fed Regist 2012;77*(170):53257–53750.
2. Rice, C. (2014, November). 5 Ways to raise HCAHPS scores via staff engagement. *HealthLeaders Media Insider,* 2014.

Resources

Hospital Consumer Assessment of Healthcare Providers and Systems—Webpage for the HCAHPS explaining the program with links to hospital ratings: http://hcahpsonline.org/ and

Hospital Compare—Medicare.gov site with specific webpage to let the consumer enter their zip code or hospital name to see how the facility rates in the various metrics for care: http://www.medicare.gov/hospitalcompare

41

Picking the Right Physician

Objective

▸ Insight and strategies to pick the right physician

Insurance

This chapter will discuss strategies to incorporate when picking a physician. The decision to choose a physician is certainly important, as your health outcome can be affected. Unfortunately, your choice may be limited. Your insurance plan may list in-network physicians or health care providers, and your choice can be limited to those listed. You may chose a health care provider out of network, but the costs you incur may not be covered by your plan. Therefore, most consumers will start their search with in-network care providers.

The best way to know which providers are in network is to call the insurance plan or obtain the list from the insurance website. Use your insurer's directory or search on its website for doctors in your network. After identifying a doctor's office a phone call to confirm that they are still in the plan may be helpful as doctors often add or drop plans.

Other Factors

Another factor to consider is the physician's hospital affiliation. If one is living in a large city, there will likely be competing health care systems and hospitals to choose from. One may value care at a particular facility, and it will be important to choose a physician that has admitting privileges or is on staff at that particular hospital.

An additional factor to consider is compatibility. More than half of Americans focus on personality when choosing a physician, according to a 2014 survey from the Associated Press and the NORC Center for Public Affairs Research. (Just 29% said the delivery of care or the patient's health outcome was most crucial.) Doctors are notorious for interrupting patients; one can ask does the doctor actually listen to my concerns? Are my questions answered? Was my diagnosis adequately explained to me? Was the future care plan presented? Some physicians may be more personable than others and patients may feel more comfortable with the more personable ones.

Another factor that may impact choosing a physician is availability. It may take weeks or months to be seen by a doctor, and extended wait times can certainly influence one's decision when picking a doctor. The office staff can also provide clues as to how the practice runs. The staff will have more interaction with patients than the physician; a friendly, respectful, and efficient staff can be invaluable.

Some physicians may be more advanced with technology than others. Does the doctor have electronic records that are accessible? Electronic health records lets your doctor track your medical history, share info with specialists, and monitor all of your drugs. Other providers may also have a patient portal, which is a secured website that gives you access to your health information. Some portals may also allow you to make your appointments, review lab results, request prescription refills, and e-mail questions to your doctor.

Be aware of red flags. Such concerns include malpractice claims and disciplinary actions. Even good doctors can get sued once or twice. Common reasons for being disciplined include substance abuse and inappropriate sexual behavior, though it can be hard to know exactly why a doctor was sanctioned. Most states let doctors practice while they receive treatment. This information may be available on the states medical websites.

Board Certification

Board certification is considered the "gold standard." Being certified through the American Board of Medical Specialties (ABMS) means a doctor has earned a medical degree from a qualified medical school, completed three to seven years of accredited residency training, is licensed by a state medical board, and has passed one or more exams administered by a member of the ABMS. To maintain the certification, the doctor is also participating in a continuing education program. *Board eligible* means that the physician has completed all components of the process, but has not taken and passed the examination. Board eligible is a common status for physicians who have very recently completed a residency program and who have not taken their examination. The examinations are usually offered once a year.

Results

One chooses a physician to manage their medical conditions and maximize their outcomes. Most businesses are results driven. If you went to a restaurant and did not enjoy the meal, would you go back? The same thinking should apply with your health care provider. It is important to ask yourself, am I getting better? If the answer is no, then you may wish to obtain a second opinion from another physician. It is concerning if your physician or health care provider is offended by letting them know you are planning to seek a second opinion. In cases where elective surgery is recommended (not life threatening conditions or urgent surgery) a second opinion should be sought.

Websites

The Internet has websites available for consumers. The sites can be helpful, but sites and content should be approached with caution. There are sites that list the doctor's education, training, and areas of expertise. This is objective information. In addition, any sanctions, malpractice claims, and insurance plans accepted by the physician are equally valuable information. Subjective information including patient satisfaction and ratings will also appear.

Healthgrades.com is a site that includes information on education, affiliated hospitals (and ratings on the hospital itself), sanctions, malpractice claims and board actions, office locations, and insurance plans. The site will also include additional information on patient satisfaction and wait times. The link is http://www.healthgrades.com/.

Another site is Vitals.com. This site can assist in finding doctors by their specialty, the patient's condition, and insurance plan. The site also includes information regarding the physician's awards, expertise, hospital affiliations, and insurance plans, as well as patient ratings. There's also a patient-comment section. The link is http://www.vitals.com/.

The *U.S. News & World Report* site offers no ratings of doctors, but it can be a very helpful site when choosing a physician. The site contains information on the physician's education, training, years in practice, hospital affiliations, certification, licensure, insurance plans, publications, and awards. The link for the site is http://health.usnews.com/doctors.

Online Resources

Caution should be exercised for the subjective information on the sites. This information may not be accurate. Anyone can access and submit a physician rating online. There is currently no way to validate the patient comments or rating sections on the sites. A very unhappy patient or a competing provider can leave fictitious comments or low ratings to adversely affect a physician. Conversely, physicians or their staff can submit very positive comments in an effort to improve patient recruitment. The internal hospital ratings of providers avoid this potential problem by offering surveys only to treated patients and are usually then compiled by a private third-party company.

It is probably best to review and emphasize a prospective physician's education, training, and certifications. Less emphasis should be placed on the subjective measures, although a review of them may give the patient a better idea of what to expect with the prospective physician.

NEED TO KNOW

When one chooses a physician, there are generally three different categories to choose from: academic, hospital employed, and private practice. The academic physician is on staff at a medical school and may also teach. Academic physicians are attuned to the latest treatments and may offer very specialized care. The academic physician will also work as part of a team, which may involve having the patient initially seen by a medical student, resident, or fellow. The learner will then present the patient's case to the academic physician (attending) for discussion. Some patients may not wish to be seen by students or residents, as this can add to the length of the visit, but other patients enjoy this detailed visit. The hospital-employed physician works for the hospital and may or may not be associated with a teaching program. This may appeal to patients, since employed physicians work in large groups and this may enable all of their records, studies, and lab results to be accessible by all of their treating physicians. The private practice physician can appeal to patients who value the physician's experience. The physician's office may have more convenient hours, access, and parking. The patient will generally not be seen by a student or physician in training. The private practice physician gets paid by what he or she does and may be more inclined to operate or perform procedures.

Resources

Healthgrades—Website that allows consumers to identify a physician by specialty or location, site also provides education, experience, certification, and patient feedback: http://www.healthgrades.com/

Vitals—Webpage that allows consumers to search a location for a physician, this site also provides information on the physician's address, education, reviews, and participating insurance plans: http://www.vitals.com/

U.S. News & World Report—Link for physician information website that provides contact information, insurance, education, and experiences for the physician: http://health.usnews.com/doctors